'All too easily many assum̲ ̲
term steady decline. Jenni̲ ̲
Whether through her own̲ , she op̲ ̲ ̲
our eyes to everyday life with dementia. How, in so many ways, we
can make life better or, sadly how, sometimes inadvertently, we can
compound the difficulties that inevitably come when living each day
with dementia. Her own gruelling journey to get a diagnosis, even as
a GP, is a wake-up call to the NHS. The anchor of faith will resonate
with many, as will the need for faith groups to embrace, not exile,
those in their community with dementia. We should all read and
learn from Jennifer and turn that learning into action.'

Jeremy Hughes, Chief Executive, Alzheimer's Society

'Tragically, Dr Bute's journey as a person with dementia began while
she was at the height of her professional powers, with her effective-
ness as a leading GP benefiting patients across the region. That she has
been able to use her doctor's knowledge and her patient experience
to help other sufferers is testament to both her inner fortitude and
dedication to her medical calling. The observant physician shines
through in Dr Bute's book, while her practical advice reveals the
resourcefulness of an inventor. In this formidable brain, Alzheimer's
disease has surely met one of its toughest ever adversaries!'

Peter Garrard, Professor of Neurology,
Neuroscience Research Centre, St George's,
University of London

'This unique monograph by Dr Jennifer Bute, a Christian medic
diagnosed with dementia a decade ago, is a "must read", especially
by the leadership and membership of every church family, for whom
it delivers exceptional insight and practical instruction and presents
a wake-up call to radical Christian rethinking, inclusiveness and
example. Jennifer's story is presented in a way that is autobiographically
detailed, open and deeply personal, freely professing the providence
and love of God throughout, but also providing sustained professional
insight, contemporary knowledge and analysis set to dispel the wide-
spread ignorance, stereotyping, "labelling", prejudice and reticence
still surrounding this highly variable cause of neurological disability.'

Professor Cameron G. Swift, PhD FRCP FRCPI,
King's College School of Medicine,
Clinical Age Research Unit

'Writing about personal experiences of adversity can be inspirational or practical. This short book has managed to be both. Some of Jennifer's suggestions for responding to the distress arising from dementia seem at first glance as though they should be obvious. Yet they are often forgotten in the frustration of dealing with someone's failing memory in a fast-moving world. Other observations shine a new light into the world of declining cognitive function. Jennifer has effectively used her skills as a doctor and teacher to provide insights that will be invaluable to anyone who comes into contact with someone with dementia.'

Derek Waller, Consultant Physician, Deputy Medical Director and Clinical IT Lead, University Hospital Southampton NHS Foundation Trust.

'Dr Jennifer Bute's beautifully written memoir is an absolute joy to read. A frank, tender and inspiring account of her life from childhood through her diagnosis with young-onset dementia, the book uses personal stories and simple examples to describe how to live well and productively with dementia. Dr Bute's deep faith, training as a physician and unfailingly positive attitude together add a unique perspective to this wonderful resource. Highly recommended for care partners and people living with dementia alike!'

Susan Macaulay, author, blogger, dementia care advocate http://myalzheimersstory.com

'The words "glorious opportunity" and "dementia" don't sit easily together, yet somehow listening to Jennifer's story they make perfect sense. Since her diagnosis with young-onset dementia a decade ago, she has given hope to thousands with the condition, and their carers, not merely by her insightful coping strategies but also by showing us a new perspective. For Jennifer, "glorious opportunity" has less to do with the power of positive thinking; rather, it is an expression of her faith in the power of Christ in all of life's circumstances.'

Chris Halls, Lecturer in Theology at Formission College and South West Ministry Training Course, member of the University of Exeter's multifaith Chaplaincy team

'I am very happy to endorse this book because it will offer hope to many carers and patients. It is precisely because the individual experience of Alzheimer's can be so very different that there will be something in this book which will be helpful to all, but on different levels.'

Vic Jacopson MBE, international evangelist and co-founder of Hope Now International Ministries

'It has long been a privilege to count Jennifer Bute among my friends. She is a remarkable woman and this has never been more evident than the way in which she has faced her life with young-onset dementia. With self-deprecating humour and a touching vulnerability, Jennifer tells her story in a way that will inspire and help those who are dealing with dementia themselves or in the lives of others. Central to the story is Jennifer's very practical Christian faith. She has placed her trust in God and she sees his hand at work in situations where many of us might be tempted to despair. There is an awful lot packed into a few pages.'

Eddie Arthur, missionary, theologian and former director of Wycliffe Bible Translators UK

'Jennifer's passion and down-to-earth approach to dementia gives people with dementia and their families a positive view of life. Jennifer is an extraordinary person with an interesting life history, but the book is much more than her personal story. Since being diagnosed with young-onset dementia in 2009, she's become an expert in understanding and coping with dementia. This book contains guidance and principles, together with examples of how they work and real-life stories that will help individuals and groups to gain a positive view of life with dementia. Jennifer's book provides the reader with an insider's story, with creative options that have the potential to open up new ways of working in partnership in the world of dementia.'

Ian Kenneth Grant Sherriff, Academic Partnership Lead for Dementia, Peninsula School of Medicine and Dentistry

'It has been an honour to have been asked to write a commendation for this wonderful book, especially as I have known Jennifer personally since 2012. In many ways we have travelled a similar journey – me as a retired nurse, Jennifer as a retired medical doctor and both living positively with dementia. Referring to the film *Close Encounters of the Third Kind* resonated deeply with me: dementia is definitely a third kind of "encounter" with life! It is clear Jennifer's faith has sustained her ability to grow and blossom into a fuller human being alongside dementia. This book speaks to your heart, to your soul and, most of all, is a tribute to Jennifer and to seeing hope in the face of dementia.'

Kate Swaffer, Chair, CEO and Co-founder,
Dementia Alliance International
www.dementiaallianceinternational.org

'Dr Jennifer Bute's Christian faith and her 25 years as a GP come together in her book, *Dementia from the Inside*, in which she tells her personal story and reveals (from the advantage of her medical viewpoint) what it's like to live with this feared condition. Far from being overwhelmed by her diagnosis, she sees it as a glorious opportunity to inform others. We learn of the Japanese memory groups she leads to "stretch the brain"; of her belief that, with the right support and understanding, people with dementia can be enabled, not disabled. The book also delivers some universal truths – not least that to be dementia-friendly is simply to be friendly, to be thoughtful and kind.'

Pippa Kelly, dementia writer, author and speaker

'Jennifer Bute is one of the most precious gems that I have discovered during the many years I have been involved in the international dementia community. Not only is Jennifer a physician, she has now found herself diagnosed with dementia, giving her a rare perspective indeed. I have always believed and repeatedly said, "Those living with dementia are the true experts; we just need to listen." Jennifer not only echoes this, her life demonstrates it. The education I have received from Jennifer Bute I could never have been taught in any school or university on the planet.'

Gary Joseph LeBlanc, founder, Dementia Mentors
www.dementiamentors.org

'This is a rare insight into dementia by an experienced clinician who has been living with the condition for many years. Jennifer's story, told with the strong core of her faith in God and with clarity and simplicity, starts as an autobiography and then details the early onset of symptoms, the decline of function and the variability of the condition. She says there are always reasons why people with dementia behave in the way they do, and that when facts are forgotten, feelings remain. We all have much to learn from her!'

Professor Kamila Hawthorne MBE MD FRCGP FRCP FAcadMEd, Vice Chair (Professional Development), Royal College of General Practitioners

'*Dementia from the Inside* is an inspirational and reflective piece of work by Dr Jennifer Bute. In this book, Jennifer openly shares experiences from her life before and after her diagnosis of dementia, and offers insight, support, hope and words of wisdom to those either living with or supporting people living with dementia.'

Jacqui Ramus, Dementia Lead, St Monica Trust

'Jennifer and I have worked alongside each other at a number of events. I am so pleased that she has decided to share her story in a book. Jennifer openly uses her own history, personal experiences and insight interwoven with her faith, to offer hope to people affected by dementia.'

Hazel Tillman, Services Manager, Alzheimer's Society, North Somerset

'*Dementia from the Inside* is written with such clarity, gentleness and humanity that it can only inspire the reader to both a greater understanding of dementia and a greater sense of hopefulness for all those affected by it. Full of authoritative insider understanding, Bute's book offers valuable insights and practical tips that will benefit all those whose lives are touched by dementia. I can highly recommend it!'

Martin Brunet, GP, Binscombe Medical Centre, Godalming, and GP Programme Director, Guildford GP Training Scheme

'This is a "must read" for any family with a member who has dementia. Dr Jennifer Bute helps the reader to understand that, when someone has dementia, the real person is still there, even when he or she finds it hard to communicate. Using personal illustrations and practical guidance, she shows how families and communities can reach that person, affirm their worth and enable them to thrive. Particularly encouraging is Dr Bute's application of the research of the Japanese neuroscientist, Professor Kawashima, which demonstrates that a combination of mental exercises, within a social context, can stimulate the brain's natural neuroplasticity to make new connections and restore some functionality. The very fact that it is written by Dr Bute almost ten years after her own diagnosis is, in itself, a demonstration that it is possible to live well with dementia.'

Nick Pollard, Family Mental Wealth Limited

'Jennifer's aims are to help people who are living with dementia, to give hope to those who are with them on the dementia journey and in all that to give glory to God. This book achieves those aims and more. It gave me, someone who is not living with dementia, a fresh understanding of how God loves the total "me": not my intellect or lack thereof; not my skills or lack thereof; nor my cleverness or lack thereof etc. Jennifer has an extra-ordinary story, but through these pages she reminds us that it's the story of an extra-ordinary God whose arms uphold us "while I swayed, weak, trembling and alone". That is why I cannot commend this book highly enough!'

Stephen Hammersley CBE, CEO Pilgrims' Friend Society

'It is profoundly moving to read Jennifer's account of her changing relationship with dementia – from the observer perspective of a doctor to the insider perspective of living with it. This is not ultimately because it is a story about loss – though it is partly that – but because it is a story about unexpected gain. In a world where people fear dementia, it is hugely encouraging to read Jennifer's testimony of God enriching her life through it. This book is also very practical, giving me new understanding for those with dementia and insights into how to interact helpfully with them.'

Tony Watkins helps Christian leaders relate media and the Bible through his research, writing and teaching.

'Few people who receive a diagnosis of Alzheimer's would describe it as a "glorious opportunity" – fewer still actually respond to the challenge in such a way as to make that a reality. This is precisely what Jennifer Bute has done over the past ten years. *Dementia from the Inside* is an inspired and inspiring book. It is accessible, honest and informative. I am sure it will prove to be an invaluable resource to many people, their carers and health professionals for many years to come. Under God it is part of Jennifer's living legacy.'

Canon Paul Harris, writer, poet, broadcaster and priest

'I am so pleased to see this book about the life and insight of Jennifer's experiences living with dementia. I have known Jennifer for 30 years and she is my spiritual role model. This book shows a very wise, practical, smart person and how she lives with dementia. She is a great friend to many and an amazing communicator and innovator. Living with dementia in a proactive way, not giving in to problems, looking for modern solutions, shows how we must never give up and never allow the identity of the person who has dementia to be forgotten. They are still there and they still have wishes, dreams and needs. Read this book and pass it on to others.'

Dr Ros Simpson, retired GP and medical teacher,
Chair of Caraway

I would like to dedicate this book to all who have dementia and all those family, friends and professionals who walk the path with them

Dementia from the Inside

A doctor's personal journey of hope

Dr Jennifer Bute with Louise Morse

First published in Great Britain in 2018

Society for Promoting Christian Knowledge
36 Causton Street
London SW1P 4ST
www.spck.org.uk

Scripture quotations marked NIV are taken from The Holy Bible, New International
Version (Anglicized edition). Copyright © 1979, 1984, 2011 by Biblica. Used by
permission of Hodder & Stoughton Ltd, an Hachette UK company. All rights
reserved. 'NIV' is a registered trademark of Biblica. UK trademark number 1448790.

Scripture quotations marked THE MESSAGE are taken from THE MESSAGE.
Copyright © by Eugene H. Peterson 1993, 1994, 1995, 1996, 2000,
2001, 2002. Used by permission of NavPress Publishing Group.

Scripture quotation marked ESV is taken from the ESV Bible (The Holy Bible,
English Standard Version), copyright © 2001 by Crossway, a publishing
ministry of Good News Publishers. Used by permission. All rights reserved.

Scripture quotation marked NLT is taken from the Holy Bible, New Living
Translation, copyright © 1996. Used by permission of Tyndale House
Publishers, Inc., Carol Stream, Illinois 60189, USA. All rights reserved.

British Library Cataloguing-in-Publication Data
A catalogue record for this book is available from the British Library

ISBN 978–0–281–08069–4
eBook ISBN 978–0–281–08070–0

1 3 5 7 9 10 8 6 4 2

Typeset by Falcon Oast Graphic Art Limited, www.falcon.uk.com
Printed in Great Britain by Jellyfish Print Solutions

eBook by Falcon Oast Graphic Art Limited, www.falcon.uk.com

Produced on paper from sustainable forests

Contents

About the authors

Dr Jennifer Bute FRGP lives in a dementia-inclusive retirement village. Previously, she worked in Africa as a missionary doctor before working as a GP for 25 years and training medical students. She retired early, as she realized that things were not right, and was diagnosed with dementia in 2009. Since then, she has devoted her time to encouraging others and challenging how people view dementia, passionately believing that more can be done to improve both the present and the future for those living with dementia. Jennifer is in demand as a public speaker at both secular and Christian events, and appears from time to time on radio and television. Her website is www.gloriousopportunity.org.

Louise Morse is a cognitive behavioural therapist whose Master's degree examined the effects on families of caring for a loved one with dementia. She is a speaker, broadcaster and writer, and researches and writes about issues relating to old age, including dementia. Louise also works in media and external relations with the Pilgrims' Friend Society, a charity founded in 1807 to give practical and spiritual support to older people.

Preface

Poppies

Poppies bloom in land that has been savagely disturbed. They grew in abundance around the bodies of fallen soldiers in the fields during the Napoleonic wars, and later, in 1914, during the First World War. Once the conflict was over the poppy was one of the only plants to grow on the barren battlefields. A hundred years later, in a striking tribute to those who had fallen, artists Paul Cummings and Tom Piper filled the moat of the Tower of London with 888,246 ceramic poppies. Tens of thousands of people visited. Looking at the thousands of bright red poppies they will have thought not only about the soldiers who died, but the effect their sacrifice had on the lives of those who lived on after them. Their deaths meant others were able to live freely.

To me, poppies are symbols of hope, life and joy. They can grow alongside new motorways in whose uncharted territory one may feel lost; suddenly coming across poppies in the bare and bleak landscape, among the gravel and dust, can give immense joy. Most of the talks I give start with a picture of poppies, because although I talk about the facts of dealing with and describing the adversity of dementia, I am convinced that for those living with dementia there are also times of joy.

When I was asked to write about how my dementia affected my relationship with God, my first reaction was to say it was the other way around. Knowing the Lord and being kept by Him affects my life with dementia more than words can say, and probably more than I realize. It is knowing Him in my life that gives me joy. I believe that as cognition becomes limited the person with dementia becomes more aware of spiritual things, possibly because inhibitions or social assumptions are removed. My dementia has greatly deepened my relationship with God; having dementia has enriched my life.

I ask God to help me rejoice in adversity. I see rejoicing as a basic scriptural instruction and there are many physical and mental benefits from doing so. Others can see my joy, and are cheered by it. Now, living in a dementia-inclusive village, I am able to walk this path with many others and encourage them to find joy and know God's love.

The aim of this book is to help people who are living with dementia and to give hope to those who are with them on the dementia journey. It is also intended to give glory to God. Psalm 51.12 says, 'Restore to me the joy of your salvation and grant me a willing spirit, to sustain me' (NIV). Whatever our circumstances, we need to have a willing spirit to know the joy of the Lord. We can't imagine the mental agony that Jesus went through as He prayed in the garden the night He was arrested. But in His prayer (Luke 22.42) it's clear that Jesus submitted His will to the Father's plan. He endured the cross for the joy that was set before Him (Hebrews 12.2).

* * *

Some years ago, there was a famous film entitled *Close Encounters of the Third Kind*. It was written and directed by Steven Spielberg, and was about how lives were dramatically changed when humans encountered alien life forms, which were introduced gradually, accompanied by musical tones and number sequences which initially the humans did not understand. Eventually, good things emerged from it all. The encounters were first at a distance, then became closer until they became personal, a meeting of individuals, person to alien. The story sequence seems to parallel my encounters with dementia, except that I could entitle my story 'Encounters of the Fifth Kind'! Each encounter has developed my knowledge of dementia and given me an understanding of it from different perspectives.

My first encounter with dementia could be said to have happened at a distance, as an academic and a doctor. The second was closer, when my father developed vascular dementia, and I experienced it from a relative's point of view. I saw how it affected him and those around him over several years. Looking back, I only wish that I'd known then what I know now.

The third and most personal encounter began when I noticed symptoms in myself in 2004, and was eventually diagnosed in 2009. Now, living with others in a dementia-inclusive village gives me yet another perspective – a fourth encounter, as it were.

But I believe that the most important encounter, which I'm listing as the fifth but perhaps should be the first, is one that began in my early childhood. I'm one of four girls, and my mother and my father loved the Lord: many people can tell of a 'before' and an 'after' experience with God, when they ask Him into their lives as Lord and Saviour, but I don't remember a time when I didn't know Him and love Him. On occasion, when listening to others' testimonies of how they came to know Jesus with this before and after experience, I can feel left out. But not for long. I am forever grateful to my parents. Knowing the love of Jesus and the power of the Holy Spirit is my greatest help in living with my dementia.

I used to be an academic GP and later in my career became a Fellow of the Royal College of General Practitioners. Ours was then the largest practice in Southampton, with eight doctors and 14,000 patients. I became the executive partner with overall responsibility. God had given me a good brain, and my intellect was an important part of who I was, and my position as senior executive helped 'define' me. In Matthew's Gospel there is the story of the rich young man whom Jesus asked to sell all he had and follow him (Matthew 19.21). His wealth was important to him, and it defined him, but God wanted *him* and not his wealth, so He asked him to give it away. Having dementia has made me realize that God wanted *me*, and not my intellectual ability or 'position'. But it was very frightening at first. Each morning I would read these words to myself (author unknown):

> Unafraid, I face with joy the morning of each day,
> Whatever looms ahead of me along the unknown way
> My heart will sing God's praises . . .

Scripture contains reference to the 'sacrifice of praise'. Sometimes our hearts overflow with praise but at other times it is a costly choice.

* * *

It may have been partly because I was a well-qualified doctor that I struggled to obtain a diagnosis. The first neurologist I saw told me, even before I sat down, that he knew me well and there was nothing the matter with me. He did no investigations and I felt humiliated.

Two years later, I was referred to a neuropsychologist. After a two-day session, she told me that my intelligence enabled me to cover up and find unusual ways of solving problems – in other words, my coping tactics were so effective nobody would believe there was anything wrong with me.

It wasn't until 2009, when I saw a third neurologist, Dr Peter Garrard in Southampton, that I was diagnosed with young-onset dementia, thought to be Alzheimer's. My foremost feeling was one of relief. When Dr Garrard moved to London I was taken over by another Southampton neurologist who confirmed the diagnosis, and was particularly interested in my situation.

So now, I'm in the unique position of being able to share from medical and personal experience, as well as understanding something of the needs of caregivers. Living alongside one another the way we do in the retirement village allows me the privilege of being able to listen to and walk with many others on the same path.

Nothing is wasted in God's economy

The story of Hagar and Ishmael shows how our pain or distress can leave benefits for others. Hagar and her son, Ishmael, had been thrown out of their home by Sarah, with Abraham's agreement (Genesis 21). The biblical account says that Hagar wandered in the wilderness of Beersheba. She ended up in what is now known as the Valley of Baca, the Valley of Weeping, fearing she and her son would die because they had been rejected. They hadn't been able to find water and she was weeping, not wanting to watch her son die of thirst. But God saw her distress and answered her. He produced a well of water in that dry and bleak wilderness, and long after Hagar and Ishmael had left the valley the well remained and continued to sustain the life of others who travelled through it. Hagar never knew that. It is referred to in Psalm 84.6, 'when they walk through the Valley of Weeping, it will become a place of refreshing springs' (NLT).

I believe it is a great privilege for me to understand dementia 'from the inside'. I gain so much spiritually by reading the Bible from the perspective of someone with dementia. It is thrilling to see the Bible as a source of so much that is helpful in understanding and caring for people with dementia. Much of this I shall share in the following chapters, as well as all that I have learned about dementia from the inside.

The facts about dementia

There still seems to be confusion about what dementia is and what it isn't, and it would be helpful to make this clearer. In some communities, dementia is considered a part of the ageing process, but it is not an inevitable part of growing old. Most older people do not get dementia. I understand that in some ethnic groups it can still be regarded as demon possession, so it is important to make it clear that dementia results from neurological and physical damage to the brain.

The word dementia describes a set of symptoms. Memory is always affected in dementia, but it is not true that all memories are lost for ever. (We will look at that later.) Other symptoms can include difficulty in performing familiar tasks, getting lost, problems with communication, with figures, with abstract thought, seeing or hearing or smelling or feeling things that no one else does, not recognizing people, not coping with once familiar activities or previously familiar places, and emotional 'unzipping' – not being able to control one's emotions. (I find this last particularly challenging at times.)

There are said to be over 100 causes of dementia, but here, briefly, are the main ones. The commonest type is Alzheimer's disease, said to account for 60 per cent of all cases but also sometimes used as an umbrella term for other dementias. Alzheimer's disease leads to a gradual deterioration of the brain; scans show that parts of the brain will have shrunk over time.

For over 20 years the cause of Alzheimer's was thought to be the accumulation of protein deposits in the brain, which was said to cause neuronal damage – an explanation known as the 'amyloid B hypothesis'. But more and more studies (including one known as the 'Nun Study', dating back to 1986) have shown that people's brains can have quite extensive deposits without the person having any of the symptoms of dementia. For more information on this, you can Google 'Dementia: The Religious Orders Study' and 'The Nun Study'. A new research focus, examining the role of inflammation and its interaction with the brain's immune cells, was initiated early in 2017, and a new Dementia Research Institute, headed by Dutch neuroscientist Dr Bart De Strooper, is planned at University College London and in five other European centres.

The second most common type is vascular dementia, resulting from lack of oxygen caused by stroke and other brain damage. There is also Lewy body dementia, which is far more common than many realize; it is usually accompanied with severe hallucinations and often with some movement difficulties and falls, but patients can appear to be normal a good deal of the time. Other types include frontotemporal dementia, or Pick's disease, which affects personality and behaviour; posterior cortical atrophy (PCA); Parkinson's dementia, which is not uncommon; and Korsakoff's syndrome, which results from thiamine deficiency caused by heavy alcohol intake.

There are recognized risk factors. One is having elevated levels of 'bad' cholesterol, LDL, which gradually builds up in the arteries. I had inherited familial hypercholesteraemia, a condition where the body lacks the gene to remove cholesterol. I suspect that this was the cause of a transient ischaemic attack (TIA, a mini stroke lasting less than 24 hours) I suffered in 2004. My GP sent me to the TIA clinic, but I didn't stop working and, as I was not allowed to drive for a while, I did visits within walking distance of the surgery with a knapsack on my back. Then in January 2005 I had an odd experience while shopping, suddenly being completely confused, unable to talk or pack the shopping into bags at the checkout. This incident was later thought to have been another TIA. I recovered and carried on.

There is hope in dementia

The rate of new cases of dementia has been dropping steadily in developed countries for the past two decades, and in the USA and the UK it has decreased by 20 per cent (Matthews, 2016). Several factors are said to be behind the decline; better living standards, exercise, education, the importance of social interactions, and the great benefit from national investment in heart disease prevention. However, the number of cases overall has not decreased as the prevalence increases with older age and more people are living longer.

In a 35-year study by researchers at Cardiff University, 90 per cent of the men living in the Welsh valley of Caerphilly were recruited and given guidelines for healthy living, such as having regular exercise and a good diet, not smoking and moderate alcohol intake. They met for regular medical checks for a range of conditions, from heart disease to diabetes to dementia. Many likened the regular meetings for tests to a school reunion and said they felt part of a community – something which cannot always be said of those who take part in scientific studies. There were significant results among the men who stuck to the regime. They had a dramatically lower chance of developing a range of illnesses including diabetes, cancer, heart disease and dementia. Cases of dementia showed a drop of 64 per cent. Typing 'Caerphilly Cohort Study: What did we learn?' into Google brings up a BBC report about the study.

There is hope, too, from the growing understanding that the brain is not a fixed structure but is able to compensate for damaged parts by forging new neuronal circuitry. This ability of the brain to form and reorganize synaptic connections, especially in response to learning or experience or following injury, is known as 'neuroplasticity'. The online Oxford Dictionary comments, 'neuroplasticity offers real hope to everyone from stroke victims to dyslexics', and now we know that dementia can also be included in that statement.

Nowadays, after a stroke we expect recovery through active intervention, such as speech therapy and physiotherapy to improve communication and mobility, and this is because other parts of the brain that have not been damaged can be used. My family has a close friend who sustained severe brain damage from a bleed and lost his ability to talk and walk. He relearned how to talk and write. It took a long time, and the strange thing was that he went through stages of writing childishly before reaching the adult form – but he reached it.

Rehabilitation is not a word currently used in dementia, although awareness of its possibilities does seem to be growing. But for the main part, the status of rehabilitation for dementia patients is where it was with stroke patients 15 years ago. Today, after a stroke we expect some improvement, although the damage in the brain is still there – so why not in dementia?

It is important to note that for both conditions the attitude of the patient can also influence outcomes. Each case of dementia is unique, a mixture of the pathology and the individual's personality. People react differently to distressing situations, and psychologists are placing more emphasis on the need to develop resilience during our lifetimes so that we can cope better with life's challenges. Resilience means the ability to bounce back, and grows from our reactions to our experiences. In the same way our experiences with God, and our willingness to trust in Him, can greatly influence our steadiness and peace of mind, particularly in dementia. An illustration is that

David had learned that God was reliable long before he met Goliath (1 Samuel 17.34–38).

The apostle Paul didn't wake up one morning and find himself 'content'. He had some dreadful experiences to go through. Olympic winners don't wake up one morning as 'medal winners': they have had years of really tough training and inconvenience. Someone told me that the athlete Victoria Pendleton couldn't wear shoes with heels for four years. That must have been tough, saying no to something that to others seems so insignificant.

* * *

In March 2012, I was taking part in a dementia conference in London and met the Japanese neuroscientist Professor Kawashima, who presented evidence that regular reading aloud, mental arithmetic and writing (the 3 Rs, as they used to be known) stimulates brain activity, and if done regularly helps to restore much communication and independence in those with clinical dementia. Professor Kawashima's work was first published in 2003, and by 2007 showed that it was possible both to delay the progression of Alzheimer's dementia in elderly patients and to delay its onset. This was an important discovery for me, and in this book I describe how I took Kawashima's principles and adapted them for regular sessions of cognitive stimulation that I run here in my village. They're called Japanese Memory Groups (JMGs), and something like 20 residents come to them twice a week. They are companionable and enjoyable times, and everyone looks forward to them.

When I look back on my life I can see tough times and heartbreak, but I can also appreciate how God kept me through them, and used them to help me learn to rely on and trust Him. I was blessed and very privileged by having a wonderful father, who had his own tough times. As I remember how he handled it all, I've often thought how some of what he suffered perhaps was also for my benefit. He never complained or became bitter. A lemon grater helps to produce wonderful flavours and tastes, but it's not much fun for the lemon! For us to release the fragrance of Christ we often have to have grating experiences.

I've found that my dementia has opened up more opportunities than I could ever have imagined. In the following chapters I'll share some of these things, and give practical information that can help and encourage others on the dementia journey.

Acknowledgements

Dr Jennifer Bute

I would like to thank all the excellent Staff at St Monica's Trust who enable me in so many ways to live well in one of their best retirement villages.

I would also like to thank all the residents who give me so many opportunities to learn and live with daily purpose. It is a joy to live among them.

Also, I am so grateful to my family and friends, who support and encourage me and hold me to account. And, of course, Louise Morse, who is a dear friend and without whom this book could not have been written.

Most of all, thanks to my God, who is my all!

Louise Morse

'Privileged' means having special rights and advantages. That's how it has felt for me, working with Jennifer on this book. She is one of the most extraordinary people I have met. As Dr Peter Garrard noted in his commendation, she has a formidable brain, but she also has a powerful spirituality and a joy that is so infectious it is almost tangible. Her joy comes from her close walk with Jesus and this is the source of her strength. I think it is this closeness that accounts for her deep scriptural insights, one of which led a Bible scholar to say, after listening to her talking at a conference, that in one passage she had uncovered what many theologians have missed. So, my first 'thank you' is to Jennifer, for the privilege of working with you on this book.

My second 'thank you' is to those who spent time reviewing each chapter and made such valuable suggestions, including Alison and Paul, two of Jennifer's children. I'm also grateful to Janet Jacob, a psychogeriatric nurse and former home manager, Stephen Hammersley MBE, Pilgrims' Friend Society's CEO, Dr Wendy Gaskell and retired pastor and Bible scholar the Reverend Roger Hitchings.

Finally, 'thank you' too to everyone at the Pilgrims' Friend Society – you have been such an encouragement. You first came to know Jennifer as a compassionate, arresting speaker at our conferences and, from the outset, saw that her book would be an invaluable help to those who are, in one way or another, coping with dementia.

1

Places and life lessons

An elderly lady with dementia whom I visit regularly always wants to know what is going on where she used to live, almost as if she thinks she is still living there. It doesn't matter that she can't take part in any of the activities or meet any of the people. She can get agitated if she doesn't know: she feels the staff are deliberately withholding information, which of course is not true. I wonder if it is part of confirming her in her reality, which we know is important for someone with dementia who is 'time travelling': that is, at that moment she perceives herself as living in a time in the past. Another lady, who has forgotten her most recent residence and is convinced she moved from an earlier address, has also become very agitated, and I wonder if this is made worse because none of her present contacts know anything about that earlier home. In contrast, an agitated resident who was waiting for assistance asked me recently if I lived in a place many miles away and, surprisingly, I knew it well. She told me she had lived there as a child, and as I told her details about the place she settled, and was perfectly calm by the time the staff arrived.

Perhaps it is an assumption that as one's dementia progresses one no longer needs to know the details of what is going on where one once lived. It seems for some that if they don't know, it can result in feelings of rejection or agitation.

Visiting a place that was once a part of your life can evoke powerful memories, for good or ill. Before we moved to Somerset, my husband Stanley and I went on a kind of farewell holiday to the Isle of Wight, revisiting places and taking photographs to put into my memory album. It was here that I'd gone to school for the first time, so we decided to visit. To my amazement, as we walked up to the school waves of terror rolled over me, together with feelings of horror. I utterly refused to go any further or pose for a photograph. I could not get Stanley to walk away fast enough. I felt myself to be once more the little six-year-old girl sitting alone in the big empty gymnasium, terrified by stories of monsters and dragons that would devour her if she moved from the bench. I was stunned at my reaction, as I had never been aware that I had these emotions. Looking back now as an adult, I presume I'd been sent to the bench in the gym as a punishment because I'd been 'naughty'. No one would have imagined that being able to read in early childhood would lead to an experience so traumatic that the memory of it, some 60 years later, could be overwhelming in its intensity.

* * *

My very early childhood was spent in Bedfordshire. My father was a Baptist minister and we lived in the church manse. My mother was an active partner with him, and I can remember accompanying her on visits to people she was caring for, particularly those who were dying. I experienced it as something good, and not to be feared.

There were four of us children, all girls. The eldest were twins, then there was me, followed by the youngest. My sense of those years up to the age of four is one of love and security. Then our lives changed literally overnight, when my mother died suddenly one night from a coronary caused by what was found to be a hereditary condition called familial hypercholesterolaemia (extremely high cholesterol). We children were thought to be too young to go to her funeral, which I think was a mistake: just because we were so young didn't mean that we should have been completely excluded. We, too, needed some closure to her death, and the experience of being surrounded by all our aunts and uncles would have been re-assuring: instead we were taken into the care of the local social services for the day and did not meet or even see any of our relatives.

Suddenly finding himself responsible for bringing up four young girls, and without his devoted soul-mate, my father must have felt his world had fallen apart. While he put the pieces of his life back together, the twins, aged six, went to live with my mother's younger brother and his wife, as they had a daughter the same age. My younger sister and I were taken after the funeral to live with my mother's parents on the Isle of Wight.

We had very little money in those post-war days, and I don't remember any of us having toys, but we were all given a doll on the day of my mother's funeral, left for us by my mother's brother. My doll was very precious to me and I still have her photograph in my album. There were no toys in my grand-parents' home either, but they did have well-stocked bookcases. My mother had been a teacher and had taught me to read, so when I moved to my grandparents' home, as they had no children's books I read books such as Hans Andersen, Grimm's fairy tales and the Arabian Nights stories. I have always loved reading. (I used to speed-read, but now I have to read one word at a time, which can drain my energy.)

Probably because my grandparents didn't know how long I would be with them, I wasn't sent to school at the usual age of five. Eventually the local authorities became aware of me and I was sent to school at the age of six. As I mentioned earlier, I would be sent frequently to the gymnasium to sit on my own.

(In retrospect, I'm surprised at the school's inability to consider the reasons behind my probable lack of cooperation.) I suspect that it was to do with my refusal to read the class books or cooperate with the materials the teachers thought suitable for a child just starting school: after all, they thought I was a year behind. I'm sure the teachers had no idea of the consequences of their actions, but I know God didn't forget me. Looking through my memories folder recently I came across a letter sent to me when I was about four years old by my very first Sunday school teacher. She had written it just after my mother died, and in it she told me that she was praying for me. I also have a letter that she wrote to me 21 years later when I was working at Mseleni, a hospital in Zululand. How amazing that she prayed for me for all those years! I wonder if she had any idea of the consequences of those prayers. We cannot overestimate the power of prayer.

A fresh start

I am sure that when my father heard how unhappy I was in the school on the Isle of Wight he decided to come and bring me and my sisters back home in time for Christmas. Only 'home' had moved to Taplow, where he had taken up a residential post as principal of All Nations Bible College, as it was known then. The nature of his job meant that even when he was working he could be on hand for his children, and he was relatively free in the holidays. The twins were able to go to Clarendon, a boarding school in North Wales. Though I'm not sure who paid their fees – it certainly wasn't my father, as we really struggled money-wise.

It was a very happy childhood. We were much loved by our father, and he taught us to cook and clean, even if our skills were rather basic when we were little. One of my memories of those days is of us girls washing the kitchen floor dressed in our bathing costumes, amid much laughter.

I owe a lot to my wonderful father. I learned so much from how he reacted to adverse events in his life. For example, he was dismissed – we felt unfairly – from All Nations College after 12 years' excellent service. Yet he never complained or became bitter, even though it meant that we struggled because we had nowhere to live and no income. I saw amazing provisions of food and accommodation over the next three years, during which I completed my A levels and went to medical school with a full grant. While I was there I went to see the person responsible for my father's dismissal. He apologized, admitting that it had not been right, and told me he had suffered personally because of it. I was grateful for this encounter, and glad that we could both move on in a positive way of acceptance and forgiveness.

In Taplow I went to the local village school, where my reading presented teachers with no problem at all. In fact, they enlisted me to help the other children with their reading, as well as with knitting and maths, which I really enjoyed. When my younger sister needed to start school, we moved to another school which I also enjoyed and have very happy memories and feelings about. While there, when I was nine, I had a teacher who introduced me to Tolkien and the fascination of history and just the joy of learning, and I remain very grateful to her. Teachers are so important.

Looking back, I can see that from a very young age I developed a love of teaching and helping others. This set a pattern that has continued and is now part of my life with dementia: I have the privilege of engaging with other people through the Japanese Memory Groups in my retirement village in Somerset and the seminars I'm invited to take on living with dementia. It speaks to me of how God has planned our lives, and equips us with all we need to fulfil His plans.

Valuable life lessons

Eventually, my younger sister and I joined our older sisters at boarding school, thanks to the generosity of another benefactor and a county grant. Again, this was a very happy time for me. Living with others at boarding school one learns more lessons than those on the curriculum – one learns valuable life lessons. On one occasion I was given some chocolate teddy bears by one of the girls. Another girl was quite poorly and very unhappy, so I gave them to her; then I was shredded in front of the rest of the dormitory for lack of appreciation and sensitivity to the original giver. My act of self-sacrifice and generosity had back-fired. But it taught me that we need to view our actions from others' perspective as well as our own.

It was here that I learned, too, that we need not accept a lack of natural ability. I'm not particularly musical, but we were taught to play the piano. I struggled – but my father had been left a pianola with a large supply of music rolls. Wonder of wonders! I could feel the notes going up and down on the pianola as I pedalled. Much to my teacher's surprise I returned after the holidays able to play a piece I hadn't mastered during the previous term, and I was able to pass a few more of the exams, well past grades 1 to 3. We can often learn other ways to do things.

My father wrote letters to each one of us every week, and we wrote to him every Sunday afternoon. There were no social welfare benefits for families like ours in those days, and he had very little money, but at the end of term when he collected us at Euston station we would be taken to a theatre or a concert or an art gallery, even if the theatre was just showing a newsreel. The concerts were free, as were the galleries. It was a treat for us and we appreciated it. At Christmas time we would wander along Oxford Street looking in the windows of the big stores at the amazing window displays, and dream dreams.

My father remarried when I was 14, and I'm sure that his new wife was appalled at the state of our housekeeping. She had very high standards which we could never attain, but I am so grateful for the opportunity to be stretched as we tried to reach them. Where else could I have learned to work so hard? Shortly after they married the county grant was withdrawn, and I went with my younger sister to the local grammar school. It meant a walk of almost a mile downhill to the bus stop, which was good if you were late in the morning, but was a trudge uphill at the end of the day when you were tired, which wasn't so good. This may have been a hangover from the time I was eight years old and broke both the bones in my lower left leg in the school playground. I'd been told then to stop crying and walk properly, though I did have a lift home from school that day. After a dreadful night I was taken to hospital, when the now rather dislocated bones were reduced with no anaesthetic. I still remember being carried from the ambulance back to the flat at All Nations where we lived. And I remember thinking that hospitals were rather wonderful!

Heading for medicine

I was fascinated with how the body works. When I was about 16 I had acute appendicitis, and I remember the houseman explaining to me what they were going to do. I found it very interesting and was impressed that he thought I should understand. A sixth-form conference in London turned out to be a milestone in my life. It was entitled 'Mosques, Men, Magic and Medicine', and there I heard Dr Anthony Barker speak. I was so mesmerized by his talk that I bought his book, *The Man Next To Me*, which was about his work in Zululand. Dr Barker suggested that I write to him if I succeeded in my dream of being accepted to study medicine.

In our school, the careers teacher considered that girls wanting to enter medicine should do so only as nurses, so when I said I wanted to do medicine she refused to support my application to medical school. But I had an obstinate streak and said I would only apply to the school that was the last to allow girls to apply and still only allowed less than 10 per cent, so she was pretty sure I wouldn't get in. However, in 1963 I got a place at Bart's – the famous St Bartholomew's teaching hospital in London – where I was one of only nine girls among more than 100 male students.

Then I wrote to Dr Barker. He replied, in perfect italic script, inviting me to spend my 'elective' as it was called (an opportunity to take three or four months away from university to gain practical experience) at his hospital, the Charles Johnson Memorial Hospital at Nqutu in Zululand. I knew he ran the hospital with the help of a constant stream of medical students rather than pay more full-time doctors. He and his wife, also a doctor, had taken it over when it was a one-bed hut, and under his amazing dedication and passion it had grown to a modern 700-bed hospital.

I spent my three or four months there as a medical student and gained more practical experience than I could ever have done in the UK. Dr Barker was a brilliant teacher and surgeon and expected us all to work as hard as he did. He started ward rounds each morning at seven o'clock. I was also given the responsibility of lecturing the nurses in medicine in the evenings (all his nurses were trained in the hospital), so I accumulated more teaching experience.

Dr Barker had incredibly high standards, a zest for life and a love for God. He led by example and inspired all of us by his enthusiasm and dedication, and his long hours of work. He would write letters at five o'clock in the morning to medical students and doctors around the world who all (rightly) felt they were important and mattered to him and his hospital. It was there that I learned the power and importance of focusing on the individual.

The people of Zululand had amazing resilience. There was something about Africa that made me feel, when I returned home, that I'd left part of my heart there. After qualifying as a doctor and gaining more qualifications in obstetrics and senior experience in paediatrics, I went back to Africa three years later.

The sinkhole

When I was at university I fell in love with someone, and we became great friends. The years passed, we were engaged and had great plans for following God's path together in the future. One weekend, while working as a doctor in North Wales in the obstetric unit (working 120 hours a week, as we did in those days), I went to visit him. He met me off the train and asked me to return the engagement ring. The bottom of my world fell out. It was like a sinkhole taking everything with it.

The following Monday I was called into the matron's office as I was a bit 'distracted', and was told if I didn't cheer up I would be out of a job by the end of the month – and no, I couldn't cancel the two weeks' holiday booked for the honeymoon. I had no support from anyone, apart from the next day when I was thrown the keys of a large Bentley by the married doctor with whom I shared patients when one of us was off duty (I had sold my car to pay the deposit for our flat). I drove up into the Welsh mountains and walked and walked, asking God to help me think His thoughts and wanting to find His path through this devastation.

I returned wedding presents I had already received and put away my wedding dress. My male friends seemed to disappear overnight. I remember getting a lot of blame for spoilt arrangements such as booked accommodation. But in my bewilderment at God's purposes I never doubted His love and care. In the pain I found God was still there, and I tried to turn the agony into prayer and care for others. I am convinced I became a better doctor through it, and much more aware of people's inner pain. Eventually I found I was very grateful for the whole experience. When waves of loss unsettled me, I prayed (as I have done since) that 'he' would walk closer with God without me than he would ever have walked with me, and eventually when he married I prayed that he would always love his wife.

I lost our shared friends, who didn't know how to respond. Over the years I had also become very close to his mother and I needed to release her, and that was hard. A poem by Annie Johnson Flint (2016) became precious to me during those dark days of heartbreak:

> I prayed for strength and then I lost awhile
> all sense of nearness, human and divine.
> The love I leaned on failed and pierced my heart,
> the hands I clung to loosed themselves from mine.
> But while I swayed, weak, trembling and alone,
> the Everlasting Arms upheld mine own.

Years later, when I was in Africa again (and at times the only doctor for over 80 miles in all directions), I was given a clay water pot which I sent back to the UK by post. It arrived in over a hundred pieces. I glued it together again and it is a constant reminder that my life was glued back together again by God's love, mercy and grace. I am sure it has beauty only because of the shattering trauma of what happened all those years ago and the utter certainty that there is nothing in this world that can separate me from God's love (Romans 8.38).

I threw myself into my work, studying for my obstetrics

and gynaecology exams, and starting a more senior position in paediatrics. Eighteen months or so later, some married friends thought they saw an opportunity to act as matchmakers and invited me over for the weekend. But when I arrived I found, to my horror, that they had arranged to go away themselves and had invited another male friend to stay; someone who'd been a fellow student at Bart's, although we'd never been close friends. I was appalled and it's possible that he was, too. So I telephoned a friend who told me to call Stanley, someone who'd been head student at my father's college and who, they knew, was living in the area. That's what I did – I telephoned Stanley and asked if he could take me out for the day so I could escape my friends' arrangement.

After that, every weekend Stanley would travel up to North Wales to visit me, and very soon he asked me to marry him. For a very long time I was reluctant to say yes: my plan was to go back to Africa, and I told him that I would let him have an answer when I returned. But Stanley was not easily put off. Undeterred, he bought me an engagement ring, which I wouldn't wear. Eventually, when I came back from Africa, I did say yes. Perhaps because he, too, had experienced a broken engagement some years earlier, Stanley took firm hold of all the arrangements. We were married in 1972 and lived in Lyndhurst before moving to Southampton where he worked as a senior social services manager – a role that almost led to his murder.

2

Challenges and miracles

It was a measure of Stanley's determination and dogged refusal to take no for an answer that he bought a house for us in England while I was working in Africa, even before I'd agreed to marry him. He airmailed photographs to show me. He'd made money by doing up a house in Bath that he'd bought in poor condition, which is how we ended up with such a good six-bedroom house in Lyndhurst, although that also needed a great deal of renovation. But that was no problem, because Stanley was brilliant at renovating a house and fixing things.

He was also wonderful in a crisis, excelling as he did in short-term projects and relationships. We made an excellent team and it brought the best out of us both: I'd always believed that in marriage, serving together, we should be more effective than as separate individuals.

From the outset we had people living with us who needed help, both long and short term. This might include the children of people we knew whose parents were in some kind of crisis. We would also have missionaries and people engaged in numerous worthy causes come and stay for varying lengths of time. Perhaps because I'd recently returned from Africa, I was asked to help with the church's Bible study for a group called Universities International Students' Wives. It had been started by Betty Hammond, someone who later became a dear friend and almost a spiritual mum to me. I got to know women from

Africa, India and many other countries. It was clear, though, that some of the wives lacked the basic skills for looking after their homes in England – skills they hadn't needed when living in the African bush. They simply lacked experience, so some came and lived with us for a while.

We were always active members of a church, and would regularly have people around for lunch, including visitors to the church. On occasion the whole church would come over. We found ways to cook for up to 100 people, and Stanley's ingenuity excelled with an old-fashioned double-bed iron bedstead that he used as an outdoor grill. I was grateful that unlike my sisters, although I never reached cordon bleu standard, I could cook in large quantities.

* * *

When we married I knew something of Stanley's background, but I hadn't realized that he had buried so much of it. I eventually extracted the truth from those who'd known him as a child. Their accounts showed that his early years were lonely and fragmented. He'd been rejected many times by the very people who should have cared for him. His childhood memories were of being locked in the house by himself with his parents out, or if they took him with them, under a table in a pub.

During the Second World War, when he was just three years old, Stanley was evacuated from London and after various failed placements, was sent alone to Cornwall where he ended up living with a wonderful family. After the war ended they naturally assumed that the best thing for him was to be reunited with his family in London, as were hundreds of other child evacuees. It took a long time to locate his parents (who'd made no attempt to contact him) but eventually they did, and he was sent back to the East End. But nothing had changed, and Stanley longed for the family in Cornwall, and made several attempts to get back to them. Once he hitchhiked down, and they welcomed him and let him stay awhile: another time, when he was 13, he cycled all the way from London, sleeping under hedges at night. On that occasion they told him that he had to go home and not come back again. They acted out of the very best intentions, not realizing that his parents didn't want him, but Stanley felt a deep sense of rejection.

For years Stanley had carried the scars of his neglected childhood, and the effect on his personality came out in the need for the security of a stable marriage. Yet he would not talk much about those experiences, even when I showed him the information I'd gathered. Nor would he have considered counselling, because his experiences had robbed him of the ability to trust people.

A walking miracle of God's grace

He did, though, trust God. He'd come to faith while doing his National Service, and he became a walking miracle of God's grace. He was proof that no matter how awful one's past experiences, they can be used to the benefit of others. It was what motivated him to gain qualifications in mental health, nursing and social work: at the time we met he was the senior mental health welfare officer with Southampton local authority.

He showed kindness, dedication and generosity in his support for others, and his career was one of service. He wrote long letters to our children and their spouses at significant times in their lives, telling them how much they were loved. He knew he would be perfect in Heaven, and they were all aware that he cared for them deeply. In church he served wherever he was needed, as treasurer, elder, on the leadership team, editor, computer operator, maintenance man and mentor. He was especially passionate about overseas mission.

It was an incident involving the safety of young children that was to lead to his attempted murder. He'd been promoted to senior social services manager and had had to take some children from their parents for their own safety. One day, while other social workers were on a tea break in the basement, leaving Stanley's office floor relatively deserted, their angry father burst into his office and tried to strangle him. I was at home, and my dear friend, Betty, came around and asked, 'What's happened to Stanley?' I replied, 'What do you mean?' She said, 'At four o'clock I had to stop what I was doing and pray for him because I knew his life was in danger.'

When Stanley came home and told me about the attack he said that in the struggle he had glimpsed the clock briefly and noticed that it was four o'clock. At that precise moment, for no apparent reason, the man dropped his arms and backed off.

Stanley's attacker was eventually sent to prison. In those days many social workers were attacked, but the incidents weren't reported, and Stanley's boss said not to say anything about it. However, Stanley used the experience for the benefit of others. He researched and wrote guidelines on dealing with violent clients, and published the first textbook on the prevention and management of violence in social work.

* * *

Our sons Paul and David were born while we were living in Lyndhurst, from where Stanley commuted to work. After a while we decided it would be a good idea to move to Southampton. We put our house up for sale and kept it tidy for over a year, but no one showed any interest in it. After 12 months we decided that it was just too much effort to keep it continuously show ready, and took it off the market. Not long afterwards the doorbell rang and, opening the front door, I found a woman on the doorstep who said she wanted to see the house. She explained she'd been interested in it for months but had never got around to coming to see it. That morning I had just done a large wash and, this being before the days of tumble dryers, had draped washing over the banisters and over the radiators. I told her that the house wasn't on the market any more, but she said, 'Please!' and insisted on looking around. Amazingly, she bought it on the spot for the price we were asking.

We found a lovely place in Southampton near Stanley's work, with perfect schools for the children, and near the church. We had signed the contracts and made all the arrangements, including buying material for the curtains and hiring the removal van, when, to our horror, we were gazumped. We'd signed our purchaser's contract, but our vendors hadn't signed ours, and they weren't going to back down. So, there we were – committed to selling our house and moving out in two weeks' time, with no house to move into. We'd spent so long looking for the right place in Southampton that we already knew nothing else was available. We decided that we would have to look for somewhere to rent, and gave away most of our furniture.

The following Saturday we drove into Southampton, asking the Lord, 'What are we going to do?' We parked the car and Paul jumped out first. He was about four years old at the time. He ran up to a car parked near ours and said to the man standing next to it, 'We're looking for a house to put our home in!'

I dashed up after him and apologized, but the man said, 'Your son says that you're looking for a house?'

I said, 'Yes, we've sold our house, we've been gazumped, and we've got nowhere to go, and we have to move out in two weeks' time!'

To my amazement he said, 'Well, I'm an estate agent and I've just come from somewhere that could be perfect for you – how much are you hoping to pay?'

We told him the price and he said that was what the seller was expecting, and suggested that we go and see the house. He wrote the address on a piece of paper (which I still have). We had no other details and knew nothing about the house, but we drove straight there with the children. We rang the door-bell and a man opened the door, and Stanley told him, 'We've just met your estate agent and he says you want to sell your house.' At that moment his wife came up behind her husband and said, 'Oh, this is an answer to prayer!'

She asked us inside to look around, and I didn't like it at all. For a start it had bright orange cupboards in the kitchen, and the garden was a churned-up mess of mud where the couple's sons had driven their motorbikes over it. But Stanley could see its potential and he loved it; in fact, he said it was perfect. (He did a lot to it and in the end, it was a very good place to live.) So he said that we would buy it, and the man laughed, 'Didn't the estate agent tell you about the condition?' We both told him no – what was the condition? It was that we had just two weeks to move in. We looked at each other and we looked at him and we looked at his wife and said, 'We've got a removal van booked already for two weeks today.'

He was astounded. His wife told him, 'I told you God would bring me someone!' She had wanted to sell, and he didn't, and he only agreed because she nagged him, so he had insisted on what he thought was an impossible condition. Some years later we met the couple again, and she told us that her husband had become a Christian partially through that experience.

If the house had been on the open market, we probably would have been gazumped again – it was happening so frequently in those days. Only God could have arranged to put the estate agent in the car park at that time, and prompted a little boy to go up to him in the way that he did. So, we didn't have to rent or look anywhere else, although we did arrive at the house with very little basic furniture. I can remember apologizing to visitors because they would have to sit on the floor.

It was God's house and He used it amazingly. Stanley fixed it expertly. He took out the orange kitchen cupboards and gave them to some missionaries who thought they were the best thing since sliced bread! Later we added extensions. A friend who was a builder did the work and members of the family helped, including the children, as they did with everything.

God had shown us on another occasion that when we obey Him the consequences are His responsibility not ours. Early one December Stanley and I felt God telling us to invite most of the people in our street for a meal and a talk about Christmas. I wanted it to be a special meal so asked someone who was an exceptionally good cook to prepare the meal for us. She agreed, and stupidly I didn't agree a price but assured her I would pay. It was a great success and everyone was delighted. However, when the bill arrived I got a surprise. We paid it, but it meant we had no money to buy food, let alone presents for the children or their stockings, other than what we had made. (Stanley made wooden toys and I made soft toys.) Stanley also realized we wouldn't have enough at the end of the month for some of our regular outgoings, so he found a night-time job as a care companion in order to earn some extra money.

On Christmas Eve, after the children were in bed, I was upstairs asking God what to do as all I had left in the fridge was one egg and I couldn't think of anything to put in their stockings. I didn't want to be seen by the carol singers when they rang the doorbell, although I could see them from my bedroom window in the dark. After some time the bell rang again and, looking out of the window, I couldn't see anyone. It rang again so I crept downstairs, looking down the empty driveway. I opened the door and there was no one there, but on the doorstep were two large carrier bags, one full of stocking presents and one full of food fit for a king. No one in the area had any idea we were in difficulties as we had told no one, and to this day I do not know where it all came from, but it was one of the best Christmases we'd had.

*   *   *

It was after our move to Southampton that I became pregnant with our daughter, Alison. But this pregnancy was unlike either of the boys'. Looking through my records recently I came across my antenatal notes. (I'm the sort of person who keeps everything of significance!) In those days you went to your GP and he would refer you to the hospital for a check-up, and then the GP looked after you until you went in for delivery. Through almost the entire pregnancy I was ill and vomited the whole time, unable to keep anything down, not even water. I can still remember sitting in the clinic, feeling so ill and vomiting, and being admitted straight from there to hospital. I was in and out of hospital for months, on a drip in a hospital bed. On two separate occasions I was recommended to have an abortion because, I was told, my life was at risk. At one stage I weighed only 50 kg when, at the same stage with the boys, I had weighed 62 kg. (The medical term for this severe sickness during pregnancy is hyperemesis gravidarum, and women who suffer with it are usually carrying girls.)

When Alison was born she was very poorly. The scale for assessing the health of newborns is called the Apgar scale, after the anaesthesiologist, Virginia Apgar, who devised it. A baby who scores eight on this scale at birth is in good health, but Alison's score was only one. At ten minutes it's meant to be above eight, but Alison's was still only two and she was put into intensive care. She survived, but had sustained some brain irritation.

She screamed her way through life for the first two years. She slept for only two and a half hours in twenty-four, and there was nothing anyone could do to stop her crying. I was so grateful to my dear friend Betty, who took her for two hours once a week. The health visitor came around one day and suggested that we leave the baby in the bedroom while she sat with me in the kitchen. 'If you don't go up and do anything she'll stop screaming in half an hour.' So, I said, 'OK, here's a cup of coffee and a plate of biscuits and we'll sit and talk.' Two hours later, with Alison still screaming, the health visitor quietly left and never came back.

We had people staying with us who said that Alison was demon possessed, so I said, 'Fine! Please pray for her and for me!' Nothing happened, and the only time that Alison stopped screaming was when she was feeding. It helped me understand, as a doctor, how mothers could reach the stage of harming their babies – not that that excuses it. (My daughter has encouraged me to include this.)

It was a very difficult time for Stanley, because he loved babies and children and they responded warmly to him. He could always stop a baby crying – but not Alison. He seemed to feel that she was rejecting him, and as a result he would have little if anything to do with her for a very long time.

As strange as it seems, it was only when she started to take an interest in books that Alison began to improve. I was teaching her older brother, Paul, how to read, and we were reading the story of the Gingerbread Man, the children gathered around me, when Paul got stuck on a word. To my surprise David told him what the word was, and we found that he could read as well as Paul. He and Alison had been listening as I taught Paul, and Alison became interested in the books. At night she would sit in her cot, and instead of screaming she would look at books. We've talked about it since and I've asked what she was thinking at the time, but she has no recollection. My daughter is lovely now, a mother herself with a lively son and husband.

I often recite some lines from the hymn 'My God I Thank Thee', by Adelaide Proctor (1858):

I thank Thee more that all our joy
Is touched with pain,
That shadows fall on brightest hours,
That thorns remain;
So that earth's joys may be our guide
And not our chain.

I thank Thee, Lord, that Thou hast kept
The best in store;
We have enough, yet not too much
To long for more:
A yearning for a deeper peace
Not known before.

*   *   *

Life was full, but I missed my medical work, and once the children were at school I decided to go back to medicine. I'd previously been sent papers to say that if I didn't do refresher placement courses I'd have to completely retrain, as you weren't allowed to do more than five years out of medicine, so I'd done those courses and loved it. Going back into medicine wasn't easy in those days for a woman – most wanted to work part time because of family commitments – and I was the first to join the Women's Retainer Scheme in Southampton. There's a requirement after qualification for three extra years of training to become a GP, and with my time in Africa and house jobs in medicine, surgery, obstetrics, paediatrics, and so on (although I had to do refresher placements in all these), I had done the equivalent of two.

I had to persuade a local surgery to employ me for two sessions a week, where they would get one session free and the government would pay for the other. So, I got my two sessions a week as a maternity leave locum, except that the surgery needed three sessions a week. So I did a third one free, and worked like that for six months because I knew it was the only way to get on the ladder. I was then able to do my official trainee year in the nearest surgery to where I lived (which was a miracle in itself) and I took my membership exams of the Royal College of General Practitioners (MRCGP) at about the end of that time.

When I'd completed the training I was able to think about a permanent position and was invited to visit the Chessel Practice in Southampton. While they were showing me around, one of the doctors said they'd like me to join them. 'Are you offering me a job?' I asked, and he said yes. Surprised, I replied, 'But you haven't seen my CV!' He said, 'We know enough about you, and we are perfectly happy with you.'

They were flexible about my hours, which was good because Stanley had said that I could only work as a doctor if nothing changed in the home. So I would take the children to school and then go on to the surgery, come back in the afternoon and collect the children from school, and when Stanley came home I would go back for the evening surgery. I would get home from evening surgery at seven o'clock (unless I was late with visits) and then had to make the evening meal. If I had not been called out too often during the night, I would leave a meal in the oven before I went to work in the morning.

I had to take my thoughts of unreasonableness to God, knowing that Stanley did love me but that was just how he was. The poem 'Love ever gives' (John Oxenham, 1852–1941) was a strength and comfort to me at those times, and I would recite it to myself:

> Love ever gives,
> Forgives – outlives,
> And ever stands
> With open hands.
> And, while it lives,
> It gives.
> For this is Love's prerogative –
> To give – and give – and give.

I was so grateful for all I'd learned from my past, including the ability to understand families in ways I would not have otherwise known: grateful, too, for other experiences, which helped me understand patients' situations in ways I could not have even imagined.

I worked in general practice for 25 years, and in 2007 I was the first woman in Hampshire to become a Fellow of the Royal College.

*   *   *

In 1991, along with many others, Stanley was made redundant from Hampshire social services. It was totally unexpected. Although everyone was aware the redundancies were being planned, he was a leader in work on the prevention and management of violence in social work and was highly regarded.

He was asked by Vic Jacopson, the author and evangelist, to help arrange – together with the astronaut James Irwin – a large Christian outreach in Czechoslovakia. Communism had just fallen, so suddenly outreaches like this could be set up openly. It was a huge exercise, involving hiring the main stadium, and someone was needed to run the whole thing. Stanley was that kind of person and he went out to do it. God blessed it and it was a success, and a good experience for Stanley. It was the start of many short-term projects overseas with Christian organizations. Eventually he joined Tearfund to work with its disaster relief team in different locations around the world, which took him away from home for months on end. As well as looking after the house and the big garden, I was a full-time doctor raising three teenagers while leading a home group and running a youth club, so Stanley's absences were not easy for me. But I'd learned from the apostle Paul that if we accept God's gift to us with both hands, with enthusiasm and joy, He can show his glory. God's gift in this instance was Stanley's absence, even if it was an unwanted present!

In 2001 I returned to Mseleni in Africa, after an absence of 30 years, for a sabbatical. I was the only doctor in outpatients and casualty, seeing hundreds of patients a day, and I often felt out of my depth. It was a challenging time, and it was only possible to cope by learning to live each day in God's strength.

Stanley and I had thought of serving God in Africa once I retired, but the onset of dementia changed our plans and our whole lives. Still, I am convinced that nothing is wasted in God's economy. My dementia would turn out to be a glorious opportunity which would help people all over the world. As a doctor, I had seen patients diagnosed with dementia and had been responsible for their care, but I had no idea that I knew so little about it and what could be done to help. I could never have imagined that getting a diagnosis for myself would take years, and be so difficult and emotionally painful.

3

Difficulty getting a diagnosis

After the children grew up and began to leave home, I went from being part time to a full-time GP at the Chessel surgery, where I had become the executive partner. We had excellent staff, many of whom I am still in contact with. I loved my work and my patients and knew their stories and home situations over several generations. It was a privilege to see the inside of so many people's lives and walk the path with them. I loved my patients, and as they came in through the door, I would silently lift each one to God.

In my social circle there were several Christians who insisted that I should be handing out Christian tracts at the surgery, yet this would have been an abuse of professional privilege. After one bruising encounter I spoke to God about it. The very first patient at my next surgery asked me, 'How do I become a Christian?' I enquired why he was asking, and he said, 'I just know God is important to you.' It would have been inappropriate for me to use surgery time to answer his question, so I gave him the details of someone else to contact. It did make my day though!

There was very little training in dementia for doctors in those days: things have changed so much in the last ten years. Often, where there was a diagnosis it was just 'senile dementia' (an appalling term) and nothing was done apart from the provision of day centres, which were more a 'babysitting' service to allow relatives to have a break than a benefit to the person with dementia. When my father developed vascular dementia, he attended a day centre where the staff, rather than finding out what mattered to him, seemed to be more concerned with 'occupation', providing activities such as jigsaws, which were never a favourite with him. When he went 'wandering', as they called it, he would very likely be found in the library, as he loved books and it was his comfort zone. Knowing what I do now, I would have shown him photographs around his room or picked up objects and talked about the memories associated with them, rather than trying to get him to understand things, which I realize now he was unable to do. But he still knew who God was and could pray fervently, even when he no longer knew who I was. I put together a book of letters written by people who were still alive and who had known him in his earlier years and in his professional life, and this was a great source of comfort to him. This was long before a 'Life Book' or a book of memories had been thought of.

Looking back on those days, I feel sad that I was unable to help my patients with dementia more; I couldn't improve things as I would do now. Each person with dementia is different, but the same principles apply to all. I strongly believe that care of those with dementia can be more proactive than is usually the case, and that enabling people with dementia to continue to take part in what is familiar to them is extremely important.

It took me longer to recognize dementia in my patients then than it would now. I remember a patient arriving late for her appointment and saying that she couldn't find the surgery, as we had moved; it wasn't true, but only later did I realize that she had dementia. Another patient missed an appointment completely and, when I telephoned, he told me the surgery had burned down so he couldn't attend. Yet another came with her husband to ask for a sick note as she was due to attend a disciplinary hearing at work. The husband was doing all the talking, and she didn't look ill in any way; I sent him off to the nurse to collect a specimen bottle so that I could talk to his wife, and quickly realized that she had marked dementia. How she had managed to do a job for so long was beyond me. It is very important to educate employers and businesses so they can spot the early signs of dementia.

* * *

In 2004 I had a transient ischaemic attack, when I lost the use of my left arm for 45 minutes. It may have been caused by a build-up of cholesterol. I knew that I had familial hyper-cholesteraemia (a condition that causes extremely high cholesterol); I had been prescribed a statin several years earlier, but within a couple of months I'd put on two stone in weight – a side effect of the medication in some patients – so I stopped taking them. My GP referred me to the TIA clinic, but I continued working, visiting patients on foot while I was temporarily banned from driving.

It was shortly after the TIA that I became aware I couldn't find my way to familiar destinations, which was very frightening. I remember that feeling still: I knew those roads like the back of my hand because I had been visiting patients for nearly 25 years, yet here I was, without a clue as to how to find the branch surgery. I couldn't find patients' homes, or even my own home after work. So I bought a Satnav. At that time I knew no one else who had one, but it was a life-saver for me.

It took five years and three different neurologists before, in 2009, I received a diagnosis of what was then referred to as early-onset Alzheimer's, and is now called young-onset dementia. The first neurologist I saw was one we knew socially and, as Stanley and I walked through the door, before we had even sat down, he said, 'Lovely to see you, Jennifer and Stanley, and I can assure you there is nothing the matter with you.' I felt that he didn't want to listen to anything I had to say, or how I had been affected, and I felt utterly humiliated. I decided never again to see another neurologist and determined to find better ways of covering up and remaining safe.

The Chessel Practice was one of the largest in Southampton. Earlier in the year, before I'd seen that first neurologist, I'd felt I wasn't coping well so I stepped down as senior executive and handed the administration over to another doctor, but I continued to do everything else that a doctor does.

I set up checks on my computer, emailing myself at the end of each consultation to remind me what I had to do – write a letter, make a phone call, talk to someone and so on. When greeted enthusiastically by people I thought I didn't know, I just responded in kind. The next thing that really worried me happened during a home visit. The patient had a visitor who, when she saw me, came over and hugged me, saying brightly, 'Hello Jennifer!' Friends hug, but doctors are not hugged in the same way. We were both at a coffee morning about two weeks later and she came over to speak to me, saying, 'I was visiting my dad when I last saw you,' and the penny dropped; she was the patient's daughter, and a friend of mine.

I began to have difficulties at home, too. Stanley would find uncompleted tasks such as half-ironed shirts, or an iron I'd forgotten to switch off. Ever the expert at practical solutions, he set up a timer on the iron so that it turned itself off after an hour. I would also find food left in the microwave, and half-made marmalade. I put instruction sheets inside cupboard doors in the kitchen to remind me how to cook a meal, even though it was still often a disaster.

Then in January 2005, when out shopping, I suddenly found myself totally confused, unable to talk or bag the shopping at the checkout. This was almost certainly caused by another TIA. I managed to drive home, but when I arrived Stanley commented on my odd, slurred speech. Later that summer I couldn't recognize family members in photographs and began to have olfactory hallucinations, detecting smells that weren't there. At the time I didn't realize what they were, so I had a gas leak check done on the house, and had the drains checked at work. I could no longer lecture from memory, so I started using PowerPoint presentations to remind me what came next.

The symptoms increased. I had auditory and visual hallucinations, hearing children screaming and babies crying, and was seen holding conversations with people who weren't there. I couldn't remember my postcode or telephone number and I had to write myself detailed directions on how to make a cup of tea and put washing powder in the washing machine. Stanley would remind me to cook meals: once I cooked supper twice on the same day, and I would also cook for absent family members. When I failed to recognize my friends and neighbours out of context I didn't let them know, but I began to keep detailed notes of changes in my behaviour and abilities. I knew I had dementia.

Then, on a long-haul flight, I collapsed and needed to be met by a resuscitation team on touchdown. It turned out to be due to cardiac problems and hypotension (very low blood pressure). My cardiologist found I had a positive tilt test, which means I am likely to pass out if I stand too long, and ventricular bigeminy, when my heartbeats can double and then miss, which means my normally slow pulse can drop dramatically. Stanley got used to my being brought home by ambulance after I'd been found unconscious in the street or in a shop. This could not continue, so the cardiologist made some marked changes to my medication.

The final warning

The two things that had the profoundest impact on me were not being able to find my way anywhere and not recognizing who people were. But the defining moment that highlighted the seriousness of it for me came when I was chairing a case conference that involved professionals from different agencies, such as the police and social services. I began by welcoming everyone, then turned to the person on my right and suggested that he introduce himself because we had never met before. He said, 'But Jenny, I've known you for twenty years!' I had no idea who he was, so I pretended not to notice and went to the next person and said, 'Well, I don't know who you are!' She replied in surprise, 'What do you mean?' It was awful: I didn't know a single person in that room. I felt that this was the end. I couldn't carry on like that.

I went to see my GP. He was an excellent doctor; we served on some of the same medical committees and we knew each other well. He could see that there was something wrong, and because of the TIAs sent me back to my cardiologist (I refused to see the neurologist again). The cardiologist was Derek Waller, a respected and nationally known senior doctor; he knew me well and he realized that there was something wrong. He told me later that he knew that I had dementia, and he encouraged me to see a second neurologist. I was reluctant, not wanting to be humiliated again; however, he did persuade me.

The neurologist ordered MRI and SPECT scans and agreed that there was something the matter, but he wasn't prepared to make a diagnosis because they had no desire to lose a good doctor like me! I suppose it was a compliment, but it wasn't at all helpful. By this stage I could no longer read easily, and when a medical insurance company representative read something back to me phonetically over the phone I thought he was speaking Chinese, and completely fell apart. So I asked to be referred to a neuropsychologist.

I spent two days with the neuropsychologist, who said that my intelligence was enabling me to cover up deficiencies. She explained that I used non-verbal and contextual clues to work things out, but that there was 'something wrong' with my temporal lobes. She couldn't say if it was safe for me to continue working. Knowing that the second neurologist hadn't given me a diagnosis, she suggested I should see Dr Peter Garrard, a neurologist known for his work in young-onset dementia. On a national TV programme, he had described how he was able to identify the beginnings of dementia in famous individuals from their use of language, for instance, former Prime Minister Harold Wilson from his speeches, and writer Iris Murdoch from her writing.

Interestingly, my children say that the first thing they noticed during this time was that my vocabulary shrank, and I began to use the wrong words. My daughter Alison studied psychology at university, and was fascinated by the words I used incorrectly. On one occasion we were in our garden and I said how lovely it was to see the 'horseshoes'. What I meant was 'foxgloves'! It's now known that words are filed in our brains according to subject as well as meaning and emotion, so I had just picked the wrong ones off the shelf: 'horse' instead of 'fox', and 'shoes' instead of 'gloves'. When I use the wrong words, Alison can often tell what I am trying to say.

The diagnosis

Stanley and I went together to see Dr Garrard in 2009. Up until then Stanley had thought that I was just not trying hard enough to pull myself together, though I'd realized for several years that I had some form of dementia. Hearing Dr Garrard's

45

diagnosis was devastating for Stanley; he rarely wept, but he did on hearing it confirmed. I was relieved and not in any way overwhelmed. We both believed that how we walk with God, our heart attitude, is what matters, not what we do for Him. My heart said, 'Well Lord, here I am with Alzheimer's: I accept this as an unexpected gift from you, an opportunity to understand dementia from the inside.'

No one at the Chessel Practice had any idea of the extent of my cover-up, but I resigned from clinical work as soon as I realized that no one could say whether I was – and would continue to be – safe. My patients meant too much to me to put them at risk. I was asked to continue to do medical appraisals, although Stanley had to drive me as I could no longer find my way, yet once at the surgeries I could function perfectly well.

Dr Garrard started me on Aricept (donepezil) which caused terrible nightmares, but I found ways of coping such as taking it in the morning and having an MP3 player under my pillow at night. It's usual to start with a half dose and then, after a certain period of time, to increase to the full dose, but when my dose was increased it caused me to fall unconscious down a flight of concrete stairs the next day at Southampton hospital. This could possibly have been predicted with my slow heart rate and missed beats, as Aricept/donepezil prolongs the QT interval, meaning it can reduce one's pulse rate even further. The fall fractured the orbital ridge in my face and the bones in my lower left arm. I can remember coming round in the resuscitation room in casualty with a terrible headache, and realizing that the doctors thought the fall had rendered me unconscious rather than the other way around.

The Aricept dose was reduced, and I was started on memantine by the memory clinic. My family were amazed at my improvement over the next three months. My hallucinations stopped (which is how I came to realize what they were) and

I was able to talk lucidly again, instead of in a 'word salad' – although this can still happen if I am very tired. After a couple of years, the hallucinations returned and became worse, but because they often appear out of context – that is, when they are totally unrelated to the situation – I now recognize them for what they are. They can be particularly unpleasant during a plane flight, but I've discovered that I can cope if I concentrate on watching a film.

Medication has made a tremendous difference to me. Initially it banished the worst of the bad smells, the olfactory hallucinations (although after a time they returned with a vengeance), and it helped me regain coherent speech.

Reading is still challenging because having to read each word separately pulls it out of context and is exhausting. But each new difficulty is an opportunity to find new coping mechanisms. There are ways around problems, although I can become discouraged at times. And, as I mentioned earlier, whatever bleak situation we find ourselves in, there can be unexpected joy. In church one day I told a friend that I was unravelling and finding it hard. She said her grandmother unravelled things to make them into new things that were just as useful. This was a real encouragement to me – I felt I might still be of some use after all!

The importance of church

Church fellowships are essential for Christians. Church is not only a place of worship but of 'building one another up' and encouraging one another. At the time of my diagnosis, Stanley and I were going to a large church with four services each Sunday. I was a member of the pastoral team, and Stanley used to preach from time to time. The vicar and his wife were exceedingly supportive, but it was clear that many people knew very little about dementia. In a pastoral team meeting before my diagnosis was known someone asked whether it was worth visiting a member of the church who now had dementia, because she wouldn't remember the visit or the visitor. It was clear that they didn't understand many basic principles, and I thought I couldn't bear to be treated like that when I became worse. So I persuaded my church to let me give a talk to the pastoral and staff team. This was so well received that they asked me to have it recorded, and my son, David, set up my website, <www.gloriousopportunity.org>, where people could view it and download my leaflets, which they could adapt for their own use.

More leaflets and videos have been added as the need for information has expanded. My daughter Alison wrote a story about a dragon who developed dementia and my son and his team made it into a cartoon, with Alison providing the voice-over, to help children understand what is happening and how it can affect the family. It's available on the website with educational notes and a link to subtitles (at <www.glorious opportunity.org/thedragonstory.php>).

I feel passionately that people with dementia should be as important to church as anyone else. God sees us as complete in Christ – and we are all valuable members of His Body. Now I am asked to speak in churches around the country, helping people, including chaplains and others who minister to people with dementia, to understand it better, to see through the dementia to the person himself or herself and be better able to communicate with them. God has given me a unique advantage in being able to teach from inside dementia, so to speak, to help others who are experiencing the same.

* * *

When I could no longer manage my own house, or recognize guests who were staying with us, let alone cook for them, Stanley and I moved to Sandford Station, a place run by St Monica's Trust, that has on-site dementia care with brilliant staff and facilities. That was in April 2011. Stanley died quite suddenly four months after we arrived. Poignantly, he died the week my article, 'A Patient's Journey: Dementia with cardiac problems', was published in the *British Medical Journal* (Bute, 2011), so Stanley, who had always been my editor and supporter, never saw it. In the space of ten days, he went from being someone who was healthy and on no medication, to being on life support in intensive care. It came out of nowhere: he suddenly developed a debilitating headache, with deafness in his right ear, pain in his right eye, nausea and increasing confusion. I had no idea as to the diagnosis but recognized it as life-threatening.

Getting an appointment with the local GP was well-nigh impossible, and when we did see one we were told to come back in three weeks as the GP was going on holiday (by which time Stanley was dead). We visited opticians, nurses and the eye hospital, who said he needed a CT scan. The radiologist technician spotted an anomaly, and called the radiologist consultant, who said it was only an old injury. I pointed out that Stanley had never had a head injury, but was told that because I had dementia, my memory was unreliable. We even went to A&E and the staff were brilliant, but the medical team had written in their notes, 'Stress, wife has dementia', and when we attended a second time they declined to come to A&E and see him. I wanted Stanley sent to Frenchay Neurology Hospital, who were willing to receive him, but they understandably needed a referral from the medical team who, based on their 'Stress . . .' assessment, refused to give it.

Part of my subsequent pain was guilt as to whether my diagnosis of dementia had contributed to his death, as the professionals, knowing my diagnosis, had disbelieved me when I said his condition was life-threatening.

When he started fitting (a condition known as status epilepticus) and became unconscious, Stanley was taken by air ambulance to Frenchay hospital, where the team was absolutely wonderful. They quickly diagnosed a (very rare) sagittal sinus thrombosis. They told us that they had a new operation to remove it and if we agreed, Stanley would be their third patient: it wouldn't bring him back, but they would like to try. I realized they needed to gain experience, so I gave permission. They took out the thrombosis successfully, but it was too late. Had they been able to do it on the first or second occasion we'd sought treatment, Stanley might still be here.

Events that unfolded afterwards included an investigation that revealed multiple failings at the other hospital. I still have a letter they wrote, with unreserved apologies, describing the positive changes that were being made as a consequence. A doctor asked if I was going to sue, but that would have altered nothing and would have taken much-needed money away from other NHS patients' care. Later, the team at Frenchay hospital published an article about Stanley's case which helped the other hospital's radiologist consultant recognize his contribution to the situation. We need to learn from our mistakes.

It was a very traumatic time. The last words Stanley said to me, with the family all around, were, 'I love you, and I always have.' In his eulogy at the funeral, Paul remarked on how his father had used his own tough experiences to help others, saying, 'In this he was helped by his Christian faith and his marriage to Mum.' Even in his death Stanley helped others, as his organs, all healthy, were donated for transplant.

Life without Stanley has taken a turn I could never have envisaged. I'm so glad that I live here, at Sandford Station. It took a while to get used to doing things on my own, even going to the restaurant, when we used to always go together. But with God's help I've learned, although I still find it difficult to go alone. I'm able to gain so much from talking with other people and their carers, listening to their stories, encouraging them and helping them understand some of their behaviours.

I've been asked to do staff training locally, and speak to different groups of carers further afield. People come from far and wide to talk to me about various issues, and I've taken part in radio and television programmes. As well as talking in churches, I'm also invited to speak at numerous conferences, including those for doctors and other medical professionals. Once I'd stopped driving Stanley used to take me, then after his death I travelled alone, by bus or train, but these days I will only travel when someone can accompany me, or transport is provided door-to-door. This is because of two frightening incidents when I only coped because God sent an angel to rescue me, each with a distinct authority and uniquely suited to the different circumstances.

4

Living and learning with dementia

We commonly find ourselves not knowing how to relate to people in certain situations, in cases of bereavement for example. It is the same with dementia; people have told me how others will avoid them because they don't know what to do or say. So I have written leaflets for my friends and acquaintances and a special leaflet for my close family.

The first small leaflet I wrote explained that I'd been diagnosed with Alzheimer's dementia, a condition that I'd been able to hide for some time, 'But now I often struggle to find the right words and often I do not know who people are, and get lost easily . . . In a large group I tend to get confused and forget what I am meant to be doing, or where I was sitting.' It included simple suggestions, such as, 'If I don't recognize you, please remind me who you are, and in what context I know you, and if necessary give me additional clues,' adding, 'If I look lost or bewildered, I probably am. Please help me, if possible, or direct me to a safe place or contact (name of person) on (telephone number).' In the leaflet I explained that some days I can communicate more easily than others and can talk quite coherently. I tend to be at my best in the mornings.

On the back of the leaflet was an important part of the message, which read:

> It can be a positive journey. It appears that the spiritual being remains true to the end and does not degenerate in the same way as the brain.

> So I can still show love and care. I will still be able to pray and be
> sure of the future. In Heaven there will be no tears or sorrow for you
> or me.

The leaflet also carried my email address, so that people could contact me later. The Wessex Faculty Royal College of General Practitioners adopted the leaflet for adaptation by any GP.

After the diagnosis I was amazed to find that there was no help or support available. I read every book in the local libraries about dementia. Stanley and I weren't sure who to contact, but eventually we phoned the local Alzheimer's Society and were invited to the under-65s group, called Connections, where we met others with young-onset dementia. We made many friends, some of whom have stayed in touch. Surprisingly, two of the other members were from our church, Doreen and her husband Gordon. They were florists and had done the flowers for our wedding. It was only because of Gordon that Stanley agreed to attend the group.

The Connections group liked my leaflets, so when they were asked if they knew someone who could speak at the Businesswomen's Annual Meeting in Basingstoke, as the original speaker had had to withdraw, they suggested that 'Jennifer should come along and tell you about the leaflets.' Of course, I didn't confine myself to speaking about the leaflets! At that meeting there was someone from the Alzheimer's Society who thought I was quite a good speaker and invited me to speak at their conference in Bristol in May 2011. The pattern of being heard by someone at one conference and being asked by them to speak at another has grown over the years and has taken me to places all over the country, from churches to university lecture halls to the House of Lords, and more.

I love the version of Romans 12.1–2 in the Message Bible. It says:

> So here's what I want you to do, God helping you: take your everyday
> ordinary life, your sleeping, eating, going-to-work, and walking-
> around life – and place it before God as an offering. Embracing what
> God does for you is the best thing you can do for Him . . . Readily
> recognize what He wants from you, and quickly respond to it.

When we recognize what God wants from us, and respond to it,
He is committed to helping us do it. He will even send angels,
as biblical accounts clearly show. Angels do not have wings
or halos, as in popular myths, but appear as ordinary human
beings, which is how it was with my 'commanding' angel.

Guiding angels

Invitations to speak at conferences usually arrive by email, together with details about the topic, the audience, the venue,
the date and time. I'd accepted an invitation to speak to district nurses in Oxford who were to have a refresher day on
dementia. I'd spoken at this particular venue before, but on
arrival was disconcerted to find no speaker's pack available
for me. This was unusual, as the packs contain useful information about other aspects of the conference, including the
layout of the building, and about the other speakers, as well as
a programme; conference organizers usually produce a pack
for each speaker. I was shown into a large lecture theatre and
taken to a seat on the platform along with three others, but as
I looked out I was puzzled to see that instead of the audience
being mainly female (most district nurses are women), it was
full of men.

There were four speakers, including me, sitting at the table,
so I asked the person next to me if I could look at her programme. I couldn't find my name in it anywhere and began to
feel that I'd gone to the wrong place, so asked her if she could
find it. She showed me a page where my name appeared, but

not under the title of the talk that I was expecting to give. I felt myself beginning to unravel; the wrong audience . . . the wrong lecture . . .

I was to speak after the coffee break. I had sent my PowerPoint presentation in advance, as requested, so during the break I asked if I could check that it was OK in the audio-visual (A/V) system. But the person I asked responded, 'What presentation?' (When I got back home I checked and found that I had, indeed, sent it ahead.) Without the presentation in the A/V system I said that I could show it from my laptop, which I'd brought with me, but was told that I couldn't use it because everything had been set up. I protested that I couldn't give my lecture without it, particularly as it wasn't the lecture that I thought I was going to give, and as no one appeared to be willing to help, I insisted that they find an IT person to sort it out. When the IT man came in he said, 'Dr Bute, how lovely to see you! I remember the talk you gave last time – you were brilliant!' I responded, 'Thank you, I'm glad somebody knows me, because nobody else seems to!'

He said connecting into the A/V was no problem, 'You could just plug your laptop in here, you take this out there and switch this over to that . . .' But I simply couldn't remember the sequence. Then he said, 'Sorry, I can't stay to do it because I have to do the IT in another lecture hall,' and walked out. I started to cry.

So, while everyone else was watching and drinking their coffee, there I was, kneeling, trying to sort out my laptop and the projector equipment, sobbing my heart out because I didn't know what to do. Suddenly a woman arrived and said in a per-emptory manner, 'Jennifer, get up, you're coming with me.' She went to the person who'd refused to help me and commanded, in a tone that brooked no nonsense, 'You are going to sort out her computer for her.'

So we walked out, and she said, 'I'm going to get you a cup of tea.' (How did she know that my name was Jennifer, when everyone else was calling me Dr Bute, and that a cup of tea is what helps to sort me out?) She fetched my tea, and then announced, 'Now you are going into the cloakroom and you are going to wash your face, and you are going to come back into the theatre and give your lecture.' I said that I wasn't going to go back, and that I didn't know what to do, and she told me that I certainly was going to go back; that she would come with me, and would sit on the platform in my chair, while I was standing doing the lecture. 'You'll be fine,' she said.

Back in I went with this woman and, of course, everyone was waiting for me. Most of them had seen me sobbing beforehand on the platform, so I began by saying that what they'd seen was a meltdown, which happens when everything becomes too much, because I have dementia. Pointing to the woman sitting in my chair, I added, 'But somebody here has sorted me out, and has enabled me to re-engage.'

I looked at her and smiled, and continued to give a modified version of the lecture I'd intended to give to the district nurses. It went very well, and at the end I got an appreciative ovation. I turned around to speak to my rescuer, but she wasn't there. The chair was empty. I asked the people who were nearest where she had gone, and did they know who she was, but they said they had no idea, they'd never seen her before and they hadn't seen her leave. Photographs had been taken during the event, so I anticipated that I'd find her on one or two of those, but she wasn't on any of them. I asked again if anyone knew who she was, but nobody did.

When I reflect on the whole incident what strikes me most of all was her imposing, authoritative presence. She was not someone you would argue with: she was the right 'person' for the circumstances – a commanding angel!

* * *

Mostly, we communicate with words, but sometimes the way a person is dressed and behaves says it all. So it was with the 'Gothic angel' who came to my rescue on a journey that involved a train breakdown, a change of train and station, and – horror of horrors – having to navigate Birmingham's New Street station in the rush hour. The last time I had been there my son-in-law had somehow managed to find me, very distressed and wandering around in a daze, trying to find the platform for the train which obviously I had missed when I had to change trains. He had been alerted by my daughter that I hadn't arrived and had left work in Cheshire in a desperate hurry in the middle of the day, to try and find me.

People with dementia don't cope well with crowds and loud noises – they can be confusing and upsetting. This time I had been speaking at a conference and was to travel from Crewe to Bristol, and as I couldn't deal with having to change trains Alison saw me safely on to a 'through' train. We'd arranged for someone to meet me on the station at the other end.

The train set off, but in a relatively short time came a public announcement, and people started panicking. I couldn't understand the message; to me it was just words and no context. I was sitting next to a very tall girl dressed in Gothic fashion, in black from head to toe, wearing earphones. I had tried briefly to be sociable, as you do, but she wouldn't say a word. Our only communication was when I said I was going to Bristol, and she nodded, indicating that she was going there as well. Shortly after the announcement was repeated a second or third time, the train began stopping and everybody was pushing to get off. Apparently, there had been a serious incident on the line and all trains had been stopped, and we had been told to make our own arrangements to reach our destinations – something I was quite incapable of doing.

We arrived at Birmingham New Street, which was packed solid with hundreds and hundreds of anxious people, desperately trying to find other trains. Because my Gothic fellow traveller was head and shoulders above all the others (she must have been at least six foot tall) and was dressed all in black she stood out, so I could follow her – and even if she got a bit ahead I could easily catch up. So that's what I did, although she took no notice of me at all. She went all around the place, and eventually we ended up on an underground platform, where everything seemed to be absolute chaos. There were hundreds of people milling around on our platform and hundreds on the platform opposite, and the noise was unbearable. I can remember thinking that the only calm place was on the railway track – seriously! It helped me understand why people feel an urge to throw themselves on the track.

The Gothic lady just stood there, and eventually a train pulled in, but she didn't get on it, so neither did I. Then another train arrived, which was packed full to bursting. There were so many people on the train that you couldn't get any more on it, but as two people got off, she lunged forward and flung her knapsack on to the two seats they'd vacated. The knapsack burst, and the contents scattered all over the seats – including her water bottle, which leaked – so no one else could have taken them. She pushed her way through, with me sticking as close as her shadow. We were almost the only people to get off that platform and on to the train. I didn't mind the damp seat!

When we arrived in Bristol she got off and I followed her. The station was packed – there were people everywhere. I didn't know what to do, so I thought I'd better follow her. She pushed through the tightly packed crowds, me still close as her shadow, and amazingly the friend who was to meet me saw me and intervened.

I don't know what I would have done without the tall,

uncommunicative Goth! The angel at the nurses' conference changed my circumstances with her authority; this one with her appearance and attitude. Now I wouldn't dream of travelling by train unaccompanied. National Rail can arrange for you to be accompanied to your train and to be met at your destination, although only once has this worked successfully for me.

Travelling is an immense challenge for anyone with dementia, quite apart from getting lost. You can also pay for the use of the business lounge at the airport; have a friendly taxi driver for unfamiliar journeys, and always carry an explanatory card.

* * *

The conference that really made a tremendous difference, and which opened my eyes to new possibilities, was a three-day national event held at the Excel Centre in London, which I went to with my son David. I was booked to speak at a session chaired by Richard Taylor, who was living with dementia and had written a book, *Alzheimer's from the Inside Out*. When I read it, I was so impressed at the way he turned his difficulties into essays, helping others to understand. The person who spoke before me was Kate Swaffer, the co-founder (with Richard) of Dementia Alliance International (DAI). Kate had been diagnosed with young-onset dementia at the age of 49. She played a video showing what having dementia meant for her, and how she saw her future. It was very moving, but David turned to me and said, 'Let's make our own, one that's more positive.' Later, he recorded a video of me giving my view about dementia and put it on my website. It's known as the 'forest video'. Kate is an amazing woman and is a good friend of mine: it was her influence that started David helping me make videos about dementia.

It was possibly at this same conference that I first met television presenter Angela Rippon. We were to meet at other conferences and subsequently I took part in a TV programme with her called *The Truth About Dementia*. I've been involved in a number of radio and TV interviews, and I suspect it is their policy that any reference to faith is edited out, although on the Sunday following one programme, I was invited to appear on *Songs of Praise*.

The most important presentation for me at the Excel conference was given by Professor Kawashima, the neurologist I mentioned earlier, who specializes in brain function and dementia prevention. He described the system he and his colleagues at Tohoku University in Japan had developed to improve the cognitive function of dementia patients. Called 'learning therapy', the system was first tried with patients with Alzheimer's at a nursing home, over a period of six months. Their cognitive abilities were then tested. Professor Kawashima said, 'We would have been happy to see their cognitive functions maintained: instead we saw them improve' (Kawashima, 2013). Patients who did not receive learning therapy had a slight decrease in their scores. And there were other improvements in the participating patients: families and nursing staff noticed that many could communicate better, and some went from being bedridden to sitting in a wheelchair or walking. Particularly impressive was the video the professor showed at the conference of a patient aged 80, who appeared to be in a coma, simply lying in bed doing nothing. She started therapy by following Japanese characters with her eyes, and went on to sit up and speak.

The evidence impressed me so much that I asked myself, 'Why aren't we doing something like this?' I decided to set up a similar programme in my village, and developed what are now called Japanese Memory Groups (JMGs). We use the principles of the 3 Rs – reading, writing and arithmetic – but with materials more suitable for us, while keeping the Japanese principles.

It's been a continuing research and development process, learning what works best. I've produced over 100 booklets, each one containing material that is suitable for people in all stages of dementia. We started with preschool materials – after all, it was the 3 Rs – but these were not acceptable, so I went on to produce more adult versions, with different sheets of paper for people depending on what worked best at their stage. But it became too chaotic for me, so I decided to incorporate everything into one booklet. Although I did it for my own benefit, it turned out to be a great success.

A regular joke is finding 'Jennifer's deliberate mistakes' in the booklets, as I seem to consistently make mistakes in their preparation. One was a question asking what the P's stand for in '12p in a P'. The funny thing was, several others said it should be '12p in a £', which I said was, correct – and which of course others pointed out was most certainly not! We all had a good laugh about it, and that does much good.

One task was to correct a well-known proverb. A resident gave me hers to read out, which I read as 'You can take a horse to water but you cannot make it drunk'. Those on her table erupted in laughter, so I had to ensure she realized it was me they were laughing at and not her. (I had read her writing incorrectly.) They are so used to laughing at my mistakes, and I don't mind in the least: they almost seem disappointed if I don't enable a howler!

Another mistake was $12 \times ? = 122$; what I meant was $12 \times ? = 144$. It frequently seems that I am no longer able to count accurately. The arithmetic is usually very simple, although there are more difficult tests for those who like it. The benefit is the speed and the thinking about numbers, and the pleasure of completing the task, although the answer isn't what's important – it's the act of thinking with the aim of 'stretching' the brain. We have a resident who enjoys challenging everyone about 'infinity' when zeros are involved. 'Writing' might be answering a question or colouring a square – anything to get the brain to respond by using the hand. I have been asked to supply an answer book for the JMG resources on my website but it is the effort of thinking that exercises the brain, not the correctness of the answer, and I'm sure that laughter enhances the benefit.

Crosswords or sudoku, or other brain training programmes, are about getting better at a particular thing, but cognitive stimulation, as in the JMGs, is more to do with stimulating different parts of the brain in quick succession. Some of the residents even say, 'Oh, I could feel that stretching my brain!'

Before the group starts, and while people are gathering, many like to do word searches. Others like colouring in, or painting with water (Aquapaint™), or perhaps putting together cut-up proverbs. We tend to start by singing familiar songs (singing helps to tie up loose ends in the brain), and then we read a poem together. I was amazed, one day, to find a resident who never seemed to say anything, reading the poem aloud with everyone else. She was even willing to read a verse alone. I was so surprised. Then we read aloud, either individually or as a group, with lots of encouragement and appropriate affirmation.

The groups have been running for over six years now. We started with ten people and now have 30, but not everyone always remembers to come! We meet twice a week for half an hour before going into lunch. The idea is that at the end of the 30-minute session, everyone leaves with a feeling of achievement and accomplishment, smiles and warmth. There has been written evidence of increased MMSE (Mini Mental State Examination) scores and improved behaviours.

The management of the village have been sufficiently impressed about the contribution that the JMGs are making to the community that they've gone out of their way to support me. I give them the master copy of any new booklets and they will print sufficient booklets for each session. Also, Chris, one of the residents, will proofread them for me when I remember to ask him. I am so grateful for those residents who faithfully support me, as I couldn't run my groups without them.

Although the system is effective, at the heart of the Japanese Memory Groups is laughter, along with relationships and warm, social interaction. We have fun, and enable joy. And each time I am reminded afresh of the three main principles that are essential to understanding and helping people with dementia.

5

Key principles for understanding people with dementia

There are three key principles when it comes to understanding people with dementia.

1 *There is always a reason* why a person is behaving in a particular way.
2 *When facts are forgotten, feelings remain.*
3 *Familiar patterns of behaviour continue.*

Finding the reason

Seeing someone sitting comfortably and turning the pages of a newspaper is nothing out of the ordinary, as a rule – unless you know that the person in question has dementia and doesn't find it easy to read a newspaper. So when I spotted a lady whose husband had gone out sitting pretending to read a newspaper, something I had never seen her do before, I knew she was behaving differently and there had to be an underlying reason. I went over and sat with her. It's best not to ask people with dementia direct questions that involve remembering anything, but at times it is certainly appropriate to ask how someone is feeling. I smiled and said, 'I can't read the newspaper easily any more,' and, identifying with her, said that sometimes I forget what I was meant to be doing. She murmured quietly, 'Do you know where I live?' 'Yes,' I said, 'We'll go together.'

That was the reason for her behaviour, in this instance – she couldn't remember where she lived. When we arrived at her flat, she became agitated because her husband wasn't there. I felt God nudging me to get the Scripture Union CD, *Words of Peace*. She didn't like it at first, but with the third song she suddenly smiled, 'I sang that in Sunday school!' She'd never gone to church, but she insisted on keeping the CD. Older people with dementia often have memories of Sunday school, which just need to be awakened.

A few years ago, I was in hospital in the acute medical ward, along with two other patients who had dementia. One had been admitted from a care home, and had been sent in with no familiar belongings of her own. She kept troubling the staff, claiming that someone had stolen her handbag. She was very agitated, and would wander off looking for something familiar. The staff were brilliant, and someone sat with her through the night. I suggested they call the care home to bring in her handbag or some photographs, something familiar to hold. Then at lunchtime her daughter appeared in a smart business suit, with some sandwiches. The mother was delighted as they chatted together. Afterwards the daughter told the staff she couldn't see a problem, but as soon as she left the mother's agitation returned. Even people without dementia can find hospitals disorientating, but for people with dementia it's even more disturbing. The care home should have sent her in with some of her own items – and for a woman, few things are as familiar as a handbag.

There is always a reason why people with dementia have 'meltdowns'. It could be sensory overload, tiredness or simply things becoming too much. Being in hospital is top of the list: it ticks all the boxes.

Situations that trigger meltdown

I now realize that there are seven situations that can precipitate my meltdown. Although they relate to me personally, they will also apply in varying degrees to other people with dementia. I've identified them as:

- trying to cope with a task that is too complicated (for example, trying to connect my laptop to the IT system at the conference I described earlier);
- being in unfamiliar surroundings;
- travel (especially when there is chaos caused by having to change trains unexpectedly, and having to find another route);
- being unwell (having an illness);
- being in a large gathering;
- being with unfamiliar people;
- having to cope with too much noise.

Sometimes these situations can be found in church and, sadly, people with dementia often give up attending church because of their distress. I remember how dismayed I felt one day when I couldn't find my way back to my place after taking communion, because I couldn't remember where I'd been sitting. All these triggers are to do with sensory overload; pain and fear can also be contributory factors.

Triggers are also a factor in behaviour that is aptly described as 'responsive behaviour'. Responsive behaviour can occur when the person is reacting to fear, or frustration, or misperceiving the circumstances. Sometimes people with dementia will become aggressive, either verbally or physically, and it is alarming and puzzling for families when the person has never exhibited this kind of behaviour before. A wife was very cross when she saw, in a mirror, her husband kissing an old lady on the forehead, because she didn't recognize the old lady as being herself! Try to identify the triggers and avoid them, if possible. It's always best to be collaborative, rather than instructive, working *with* the person, not directing him or her.

* * *

When Stanley and I moved to Sandford we started attending a new church. After he died, I told the leaders about the possibility of my having meltdowns. One response was, 'Well, don't come to church then!' I ignored this and made sure that responsible people in the church had copies of the leaflet I'd written about meltdown, so they would be prepared. It was a good thing that I did!

One Palm Sunday the minister decided to do something quite different, which involved walking round the building with lots of noisy musical instruments. Thankfully, my meltdown was dealt with brilliantly, without causing problems to the rest of the congregation. I was taken into a side room and someone read from my 'Prayers for Tough Times' (which my previous church had asked me to compile) and provided the ubiquitous cup of tea and some soothing hymn music until I settled. They said they wouldn't have known what to do without the leaflet. The minister apologized and said he realized he should have warned me in advance. I have good friends now who take me to church, although I tend to sit at the back or near a wall and allow them to collect refreshments for me. I am confident that they will help me cope. And it is encouraging that more and more churches are taking the trouble to learn about dementia and are becoming 'dementia inclusive'.

Although I didn't see it at the time, all the triggers were present at a community barbecue to mark the opening of a new section of the residents' gardens, and to say farewell to a very popular member of staff. I'd been particularly looking forward to it and arrived early, before some of the staff, and helped by getting chairs and food and cutlery. The event was being held in a somewhat unfamiliar place with loud music and lots of people whom I didn't recognize. In addition, I was tired because the day before had been particularly draining. More and more people came, and I realized I was also seeing people who weren't there: I was having hallucinations and was heading for a meltdown. I stopped taking part, became increasingly withdrawn and eventually unresponsive, and soon had tears streaming down my face. It seemed to take ages before anyone noticed. They just carried on talking to me or expecting my help. Eventually a friend came over, linked her arm in mine and led me away saying, 'I'm going home to get my sunglasses, and you're coming with me.' She was brilliant! It was such a normal, friendly approach that I didn't feel humiliated in any way.

I had forgotten that, as it was late in the afternoon, it was the time that the energy and mood of people with dementia can take a dip, although the sun was shining brightly. This can be called sundowning. I made a video about it for my website, but it was only on reviewing it and listening to myself that I realized that this was what had happened, and that I should have either not attended the event at that time, in those circumstances, or should have set up someone to keep an eye on me to protect me from the sensory overload.

How to help someone in meltdown

Not all meltdown behaviour is like mine. The meltdown behaviour of other people with dementia reflects how they were when they were little. They will get cross or agitated, or yell or throw things, or swipe things off the table, or rock back and forth, the sort of behaviours we talk about when describing what toddlers do. But whatever the behaviour, it reflects the vulnerability of a child and calls for understanding and gentleness from others and help, in the ways I've described. More often than not, people will empathize with children but not with someone with dementia.

When I revert to childhood patterns, as people with dementia do when things become too much, I remember what Jesus said about children and the kingdom of Heaven. He said, 'I'm telling you . . . Whoever becomes simple again, like this child, will rank high in God's kingdom. What's more, when you receive the childlike on my account, it's the same as receiving me' (Matthew 18.2–5, THE MESSAGE).

There are things to do that can reassure me, and others like me with dementia who experience meltdown. If I don't know you, or have forgotten that I do, introduce yourself with some context; for example, say, 'I'm Sheila, and I help serve teas and coffees at church,' or whatever is appropriate. Please don't ask me questions: as a rule, it's never helpful to start a conversation by asking questions of people living with dementia. Then, if possible, simplify or calm my environment, and if this can't be done, take me out of it as the people in church did on Palm Sunday. Calming the environment might include making it less noisy, perhaps by turning the music down or off, or adjusting the lighting by switching more lights on, or if necessary, off – in other words, removing or reducing the sensory triggers.

If I'm confused, reassure me, but don't overwhelm me with words – show me what I should do. You might simply point to the door, hold out an arm to me and, with a smile, mime the pouring of a cup of tea. Then in a quieter, less stressful place, perhaps you could play suitable music, and talk with me about the hobbies, the passions, the subjects that meant a great deal to me earlier in my life.

What did Jesus do when the disciples had a meltdown after the resurrection when He appeared to them in the upper room? They were terrified. He reassured them by telling them to look, to touch, to find him food – familiar patterns that gave them something to do (Luke 24.36–49). When Peter was worrying how they would pay their temple tax, Jesus sent him to do something familiar – catch a fish.

When facts are forgotten, feelings remain

I found myself in conversation with Harry (not his real name) one day. He asked me, why did I bother with God? It turned out that he'd stopped going to church because of a misunderstanding and had been told that he wasn't welcome as he hadn't attended communion for over six months. He remembered those feelings of rejection. I told him that God still welcomed him, even if that particular church didn't. It was as if a burden rolled from his shoulders.

Sometimes people will say, why bother to visit someone who's forgotten who they are, or don't remember you after you've gone? Although the person may have forgotten who you are, they will remember how they feel, and visiting will evoke those good feelings, particularly when you bring warmth and love. People with dementia will enjoy your visit, even if they don't remember what they did or who it was with, so we can give them pleasure even if they forget that it was us.

Christine Bryden is an Australian lady who was diagnosed with young-onset dementia at the age of 46. Dismayed at finding no information that could help people with dementia, only their carers, she helped form the Dementia Advocacy and Support Network International (DASNI). Speaking at a conference in New Zealand she said:

> If I enjoy your visit, why must I remember it? Why must I remember who you are? Is this just to satisfy your OWN need for identity? So please allow Christ to work through you. Let me live in the present. If

I forget a pleasant memory, it does not mean that it was not important for me.

Feelings are heightened in dementia. We pick up your mood, whether you are calm or agitated. (This is known as mirroring.) Naomi was very agitated one day, and it took me ages to find out why – that her carer had turned up in the morning upset and sad because of a family crisis, and Naomi thought it must have been because of something she had done, although she couldn't remember what that might have been.

Familiar patterns of behaviour continue

When behaviour is repeated again and again, we establish a pattern that becomes embedded in our memory and is laid down in our subconscious. Our brain builds neuronal circuits that become automatic. For instance, when we are learning to drive we are conscious of every action – depressing the clutch, changing gears, signalling turns, and so on. But after a while, when we've acquired the skills and road craft, we've built neuronal circuits in our brains that are triggered automatically when we start to drive. It's the same when our route takes us through the same streets to work every morning and back every evening: after a while we say we are driving on 'automatic'. The pattern has become embedded in our subconscious. When you see people using a keyboard without looking at the keys, you're seeing the same principle in action.

You may remember the TV programme sponsored by the Alzheimer's Society, called *Barbara and Malcolm: A Love Story*. The camera crew lived with Barbara and Malcolm for several months, filming their lives and Malcolm's deepening dementia. Malcolm had been an accomplished pianist, and it was remarkable to see how even when he seemed to be 'lost' he would sit at a piano and play complicated and beautiful music.

Years of practice and performing meant that he could play on 'automatic', even when he could no longer read music. It also seemed to be comforting to him.

Another example of familiar behaviour that was also comforting, although puzzling at first, was when Frank, who'd had dementia for nearly nine years, took to rearranging the shopping on the belt at the supermarket checkout and, if his wife Linda didn't stop him in time, would surprise shoppers by rearranging their groceries too (Morse, 2010). At home, when Linda was out of the room for any length of time, Frank would move the furniture around in the sitting room, although afterwards he couldn't remember doing it. The explanation came from the job he'd had for many years. Frank had been the transport manager of a large warehouse company, where he was responsible for making sure that trucks were loaded and sent out in time to supermarkets all over the country. If a truck missed its time slot at the supermarket, the unloading bay would be taken by another and it would have to arrange another slot, so it could be a demanding and stressful job. Frank often used to help line up the consignment for loading into the trucks. In moving the furniture, he was reverting to familiar behaviour that was also comforting, or comfortable.

One day, I attended a lecture in another part of our village on dementia and memory, given by a well-known trainer. Many of the slides were dated more than ten years earlier, and there were so many that, halfway through, I began to suffer with sensory overload. I found myself disagreeing with everything that was being said and began to get agitated, but I didn't know how to leave, so I had to endure 92 minutes of non-stop talking. I was in meltdown, and I asked another resident to help me find my way out.

He took me to the door, then turned and went back in. I just stood there, as I couldn't remember how to get home, and I was about to wander off when a senior member of staff came rushing up saying I was being asked for, as someone had had a fall. He had fallen over and there was blood everywhere from a nasty deep gash in his face caused by his glasses. The emergency switched me into medical mode immediately. I examined his face and realized he needed stitches, and asked someone to take him to A&E. Once the incident was over, I reverted to not knowing where I was, or who any of the people gathered around me were. Another resident saw how I was and took charge, taking me back to my flat. This particular lady has always been able to tell if I am adrift, even if no one else is aware of it. I am very grateful to those who help me when I need it.

Coping with hallucinations

At the time of writing, there are 539,062 people in the UK who have been diagnosed with dementia (Alzheimer's Research UK). Each one is unique, and their symptoms are different, but the same principles apply to everyone, including those who have hallucinations. I believe all hallucinations come from previous memories and episodes stored in our brains that re-emerge at inappropriate times and in random order, mixed together in bizarre ways. Some of mine come from my medical experiences. Coming back in a taxi from the conference whose unsettling events I described in the last chapter, I could see my decapitated head floating upside down inside the car, bouncing off the roof or the windows, and causing me to duck as it came my way. (The increasing violence shown in films and TV programmes raises the question of the effects it will have on people who watch them now, should they develop dementia when they are older.)

Another hallucination was the swarm of bees that swirled

around my head, that I tried to get away from, batting them off as I ran. At times my olfactory (smelling) hallucinations overwhelm me and I struggle. They tend to occur during meals, which is tough. I am sure many come from my experiences in the slums of Calcutta (where I once spent a little time) or from my time in Africa. I remember, at one leaving ceremony, an African saying that they had noticed that 'smells' had never affected my relationships with them. On reflection, I can see that it was easy then; they were people in great need, and my concern and love for them would 'overwrite' the dreadful smells. But now they rise unbidden with nothing to suppress them. The smell of freshly ground coffee can overwrite them for about 20 minutes, but sometimes that's not long enough!

When I hear the phone ringing or the sound of old-fashioned typewriters next door, or even babies crying upstairs, I know it can't be real, but I still go and have a look. I've tried to overwrite these sounds by putting on some music, or by playing the keyboard or going to talk to one of the village's brilliant porters – not that they realize why!

When I feel someone tugging at my arm I try and find something for the arm to do. Or, when out walking, I suddenly feel I am walking on jagged stones and I yell out, I give my feet a firm massage. I will always try to overwrite the messages being flagged up in my brain.

Listening for the meaning behind the words

Dementia brings changes in thought patterns; thoughts often come out as words and these can be significant, expressing the person's needs or feelings, even if those needs are not easy to recognize. It's important to listen to the meaning behind the words. For example, someone might ask, 'What time is it?' when their question is really, 'What am I meant to be doing?'

Each situation is different, of course, but a helpful answer in that case might be, 'It's four o'clock and we will be having tea very soon.'

Saying 'I want to go home' (often when the person already is at home) could mean that the person isn't feeling at home; that she's not at ease within herself. When you know the person you know what will make him or her feel more comfortable and more at home. Each person is different – the answer could be making a cup of tea and biscuits, or playing his favourite music, or sitting down alongside him for a few minutes and chatting.

Miriam, a lady I visit, always asks me what I am having to eat later in the day. At first this surprised me, but now I take it as a compliment, as I discovered that providing meals for people was very important to her in the past. I've also discovered that if, when I get up to go, she asks me, 'What is happening now?' she really wants to know when she will be having her next meal, and which meal it will be. I suspect, too, that it also means she is feeling uncared for, so I tell her about the meal and reassure her as to when I will be visiting next – and she smiles again.

'The peas are green on Saturday,' I was told when I visited one of my 'regulars' recently. She didn't appear to know who I was. I thought she was being polite, trying to make conversation. I knew from experience that it didn't go down well if I explained who I was, so I sat down, smiled and said, 'Yes, they are,' and made a further comment. She replied, 'The peas are green on Saturday.'

No matter what I said, talking to her about other familiar things, the reply was always the same: a bit like a broken record. I needed to find some way to move it on, and nothing seemed to work. So I started singing a song from her childhood. To my amazement she immediately joined in and we sang it together. When we stopped she smiled at me and asked me to repeat something I had said earlier. Sometimes we need to make a detour to enable the other person to re-engage. We know singing can help to tie up the loose ends in our brains or move on the broken record!

Finding another way around is always possible. I often say, 'When the front door is shut, and the key is lost, there is usually a back door or a ladder with which to climb in the window.' Another analogy is that when a tunnel is blocked in the London Underground, you don't simply abandon your journey, you find an alternative route.

Just before my diagnosis I had an experience when a friend tapped me on the shoulder in Waitrose and said, 'Why are you ignoring me, Jennifer?'

'I don't know who you are! I've never seen you before!' I said.

She responded by telling me her name.

I looked at her. 'I've never heard of you.'

'We go to the same church, and we serve on the same team; you had tea with me last week.'

'I'm sorry, I don't remember.'

Then, because she continued to try and find clues to help me remember, after a few more minutes, it was as if the lights suddenly went on and I did remember who she was. It's a bit like adding rungs to a ladder – you add one and I step on it, and then another and another, and perhaps another, until I arrive at the place where it all makes sense.

All my experience and knowledge tell me that when someone has dementia, the real person is still there, even if trapped within a body and a condition that makes it hard for them to communicate. It gives me great joy to 'find' those who are further along the path than I am. In the next chapter I'll look at ways of reaching the person, of affirming his or her worth and enabling that person.

No matter what stage the dementia, the ability to receive and to give love never goes. I was listening to the well-known passage about love in a new translation of the Bible and I thought how relevant it was to dementia. It was 1 Corinthians 13.8–13, in The Message Bible.

> Love never dies . . . understanding will reach its limit . . . We don't yet see things clearly. We're squinting in a fog, peering through a mist. But it won't be long before the weather clears and the sun shines bright! We'll see it all then . . . But for right now, until that completeness, we have three things to do . . . Trust steadily in God, hope unswervingly, love extravagantly.

6

Don't disable – enable

Treat everyone with kindness, dignity, compassion and respect whether you think they understand or not: never underestimate the power of the mind, the importance of love and faith, and to never stop dreaming.

This is the message to the world from a young man who, for ten years, had been trapped in an unresponsive body following a short, mysterious sickness. Martin Pistorius had fallen seriously ill at the age of 12 and lost control of his body. His parents were told that he had no awareness of the world around him. For ten years he was unable to communicate and grew up with everyone around him assuming he was brain-dead. Then, a therapist saw 'a glimmer in his eye' and knew that there *was* someone alive in there. Tests showed that Martin could, in fact communicate, and it was a turning point in his life. He learned to talk with a computer-aided device, learned to drive, went to college, met a young lady and got married. He's even written a book, called *Ghost Boy.*

Martin had been lost because, until the therapist spotted the glimmer in his eye, no one had bothered to try and find him. It's the same with people with dementia who lose the ability to communicate: the assumption is that the person's brain is so damaged that they are no longer 'in there'.

Yet there is evidence that this is not true at all. It's widely known that there are times when someone with dementia who hasn't communicated for some time and seems to be 'locked in', suddenly comes back to herself with faculties that she had apparently lost. This 'reappearing' is often prompted by different stimuli, perhaps singing, or the reading of Scripture. Tom Kitwood (1997), the Alois Alzheimer Professor of Psychogerontology at Bradford University and a leading pioneer in dementia care, said that there was no medical explanation for these occurrences other than that 'even a brain which is carrying severe pathology may have more reserve and flexibility than is commonly assumed.' Whatever the medical explanation, these 'breakthroughs' show that *the person remains*, shut inside his condition and unable to 'get out'. It also underlines the importance of finding the 'back door' or the 'window' described earlier.

Very often, music that is special to the person can be an effective back door. In a YouTube video, a carer in a nursing home in the USA describes how a female resident with dementia had been unresponsive for two years, not reacting to anything they tried, barely opening her eyes. And then iPods were introduced to the home. The lady's family described the music she'd liked, and once the iPod was loaded and placed over her ears 'she started shaking her feet, she started moving her head. Her son was just amazed!' Emotion at the memory overcomes the carer so she can hardly speak.

Then the story moves to Henry, a man who had been in the nursing home for ten years, and who sat day after day, slumped over with his head down, almost mute and unable to answer the simplest questions. His daughter said that before his illness he'd always been fun-loving and singing, that 'he was always into music'. He used to quote the Bible, so the carer found Christian music for him to listen to. Neurologist Oliver Sacks is shown in the video, commenting that, 'We first see Henry inert, maybe depressed, unresponsive, and almost unalive.' Then he's given an iPod containing his favourite music. As soon as he hears the music Henry's face lights up; he begins singing and becomes animated, moving in time to the tune. Oliver Sacks comments on the lasting effect of the music; that it has had a 'quickening effect' on Henry's brain. Afterwards Henry talks movingly, saying that 'music means God, and God is love'. You can see the YouTube video by Googling 'Man in nursing home responds to music'.

Inspired by Henry's experience, the students of Lakehouse Music Academy in the USA partnered with the Alive Inside Foundation to explore the healing power of music in older people with dementia. A local TV station made a programme about their work, which you can see if you search YouTube for 'Elders with Dementia'.

I was asked to help in a new venture at church for people who lived in local care homes as some of the volunteers were a bit anxious about how they could relate to those living with dementia. I went around talking to our 'visitors' and made sure that each helper had a starting point for their chat. There was one gentleman without a visitor, sitting in a wheelchair by himself. He wasn't really saying anything, so I went over and sat with him.

'I'm Jennifer, and I hear you are in your nineties. You must have had an amazing life,' I began. He nodded. 'Well,' I said, 'perhaps you spent some of it abroad.'

He made a noise and nodded enthusiastically. 'Perhaps you even worked abroad . . .' He nodded and tried to say something, though it sounded like a grunt.

'I worked abroad,' I said, 'I was in Africa.' He became quite animated, so I continued, 'It seems you were as well – I was in Zululand nearer the south . . .' No response. 'Perhaps you were nearer the north.' There were more noises and apparent enthusiasm.

By this time everyone else in the hall was listening. 'It must have been quite an experience,' I continued. 'I was working as a doctor there.' He started waving his arms around and making attempts to say something, but I couldn't understand him. I hesitated and said, 'I once knew a doctor who worked in North Africa called Philip Rigby.'

He began beating his chest and making a loud noise that could have been 'Me, me.' I stared at him in disbelief. 'Are you the Philip Rigby I worked with at Clerkenwell Medical Mission when I was at Bart's fifty years ago?' I would never have found this out if I had not bothered with this elderly gentleman apparently abandoned in his wheelchair.

On subsequent afternoons he would sometimes be able to talk and would do his best to introduce me proudly to anyone around. On other afternoons he didn't have a clue who I was – but I always knew who he was!

Don't make the mistake that I did when visiting someone I hadn't seen for a couple of weeks, because I'd been with my family. Vera had no idea who I was when I arrived, and I knew that if I told her my name she would get angry. So I started telling her about a place I had recently visited that she also knew. All went well while we were chatting about it, until I said, 'And what have you been doing while I was away?'

How could I have been so insensitive and broken my own rules about never asking that kind of question? How was she to remember anyway? I suppose I forgot, and oh my! – the anger that erupted. But it was entirely my fault not hers. Much 'challenging behaviour' is the result of someone's inappropriate action.

Three days later I returned to find her seemingly far away, staring blankly at the TV screen, unintelligible and unable to string a sentence together. So I chatted about the weather, the picture of a member of the royal family in the newspaper, referred to the sound of church bells on the TV, laughed at a silly advert, and so on. At one point she looked up and asked, 'Have you packed up everything and made the sandwiches?' I assured her all was under control and went on chatting, removing dead flowers from her vases, which always pleases her.

Suddenly she asked, 'When are you meeting up with all your family?' I was amazed. I told her I had met them the previous week and she asked if the grandchildren were now back at school. These times of lucidity and recalled memory can be completely unexpected!

Enabling conversation

Thomas was someone I got to know, and one day I heard that he'd had a severe stroke and had been taken to hospital. He was there for a few months and on his return, I was told that it wasn't worth visiting him because he couldn't talk. Well, this was a challenge to me, so I went over to see him. He was just lying there, hardly able to move, so I went in and spoke to him. My medical background is intrinsic to who I am, so I ascertained his condition and decided a lot could be done to improve things. Physiotherapy, occupational therapy and speech therapy can all make a great difference. We were able to get physiotherapy but not speech therapy, so I did my best with the latter. You can help people to talk; you take what they can do and improve it, and move it along. I visited him regularly just to sit and talk.

He had a little movement in one arm and was eventually able to sit in a wheelchair. He is also speaking now; haltingly, but he speaks. I was aware that he was a Christian and had been active in the church, so I used to talk to him about God. After some considerable time, he moved to a different part of the country, but before he left he said to me, 'You know,

Jennifer, I've been in a spiritual wilderness these last few years.' So, I said, 'Well, what are you going to do about it then?' I was so grateful that God allowed me to know that, before he left, and I continued to pray for him.

George joined us at Sandford after having a severe stroke. When I saw him I would ask, 'How are you today?' He would raise his thumb in a positive gesture, and I would say with a grin, 'Sorry, I didn't hear that!' I would ask the question again until he replied with just something. Speech comes with practice – that's how we learn as children, and after a stroke or in other situations we might need to learn again. Those around us can contribute so much just by giving the person time.

Spending time with people with dementia not only improves their ability to communicate but contributes to their sense of well-being. Approximately 70 per cent of residents in Pilgrim Homes' care homes have dementia, and the charity has developed a method of care that involves carers interacting with individuals frequently, talking about their interests, showing pictures and other items that are relevant to them. They've called this the Hummingbird approach. It helps prevent those with dementia sinking into silence and becoming 'lost'. It's a Christian charity whose ethos springs from Matthew 25.40: 'The King will reply, "Truly I tell you, whatever you did for one of the least of these brothers and sisters of mine, you did for me"' (NIV).

A great deal can be found out without asking questions. One lady with advanced dementia, who was confined to her wheelchair, seemed quite unresponsive. Her husband was devoted to her and would wheel her around outside in the sun. I made a point of always making eye contact with her; chatting to her, smiling and holding her hand. One day I was sitting outside with the couple, chatting away to her, and she suddenly started talking. But I couldn't understand a word! I turned to her husband to say that was not what I had hoped to achieve and saw he was grinning. 'She is talking Danish,' he said, 'We met as students in Denmark.' So, then it was a matter of finding some Danish songs and stories for her to listen to.

It's love and relationships that count

Often, just coming alongside people where they are, with kindness and respect, and confirming them in their reality, helps them move into ours.

I was sitting in the lounge after our midday meal between two gentlemen who both had dementia, and commented to one how lovely it was to see his son at lunch. 'I don't have a son,' he replied. Whoops! I ignored that and mentioned his wife. 'I'm not married,' he rejoined. Ah . . . he was time travelling, back to a time before he was married.

I was born after the war, so I turned to the gentleman on the other side of me (with whom I'd had previous chats) and said, 'You have some wonderful stories to tell about the war.' Soon the two of them were reminiscing together. To my amazement, after about 15 minutes the first one turned to me and said, 'You are right, I do have a son.'

You may assume we do not remember, and often we don't, but you can never be sure what we do remember – so please never tell us lies or insist we are wrong: it won't help us!

I have just watched the film *Marjorie Prime* and found it fascinating on many levels. It's set in 2050 and is about an 80-year-old woman with dementia, who spends time talking with a holographic image of her deceased husband, Walter. She has chosen a 'young' version of Walter who has been primed with information by her son-in-law. The process is designed to help her talk and remember things from her past. She tells him her life stories and they can reminisce together.

Her carer also confides in Walter, but Marjorie's daughter refuses to acknowledge him as she dislikes that version of her dad. Walter, the hologram, becomes curious about who the real Walter was, and asks the son-in-law, eventually discovering an unmentionable family secret. Later in the film we see the mother talking to her daughter, but we realize Marjorie has died and the daughter is talking to a holographic projection of her mother to help her cope with her death. The daughter has chosen the version of her mother with dementia, which is interesting.

At the end the holographic projections of father, mother and daughter share their knowledge of the family and are surprised to find out the 'truth' and make sense of it all. The son-in-law, who was fully aware of everything, and whose worth and wisdom was unrecognized in life, is absent from the gathering.

Do we remember our version of events or someone else's? Does it matter? How can we know, if others will not talk about it? In relationships, openness and truth are important, but in the end it is love and acceptance that count.

Things that disable

Examples of remarks that are disabling for someone with dementia, even if unintentionally, are, 'What have you been doing lately?', 'I don't suppose you remember, but . . .', 'You know you're remembering that all wrong . . .', 'You've already told me that four times . . .' Questions and comments like this are unhelpful and can cause problems – and, as you know, I have been guilty myself! In the previous chapter I mentioned how important it is not to ask questions that require the person to delve into her memory, which can be unsettling and cause her to freeze; instead, ask a more present-related question, such as, 'How are you feeling?'

Jesus said, 'Here is a simple, rule-of-thumb guide for be-haviour: Ask yourself what you want people to do for you, then grab the initiative and do it for *them*' (Matthew 7.12, THE MESSAGE).

One day I had my dress on inside out, but nobody said any-thing about it until a visitor pointed it out to me. So later in the day I said to the others with a laugh, 'I was wearing my dress inside out and nobody seemed to notice!' And they said, 'Oh, we all do that!' But of course, they don't. Why didn't someone tell me I was wearing my dress inside out? It's better for people to say something is wrong, such as the inside-out dress, and to laugh with me. That's what my family would do! No one likes being laughed *at*, but telling someone that something is wrong and laughing *with* them about it has the effect of making them feel accepted as a member of the group. Not telling them and letting them discover afterwards makes them feel the oppos-ite; that they're not part of the group, they're not important enough to help put things right.

I remember the first time I was given a banana. I had no idea how to eat it. Should I peel it? I remember the feeling now, when I see someone with dementia not knowing how to eat a certain type of food or how to 'open' it, and uncertain as to whether they should use a knife and fork or a spoon. So what did I do with my banana? I watched how others ate it and copied them, and this is what we do now. If there is someone else doing something, we can copy them. A short while ago a lady with dementia was given soup to eat as she had been poorly, but she was sitting at a table with others eating meat and two veg so she picked up her knife and fork to eat her soup. This was considered an indication of how bad her condition was, rather than a reminder to the people around her that she needed help. I wanted to order a bowl of soup and go and sit at her table, but it wasn't possible in that instance.

My children are often abroad, and I once had some presents to send to one of them, which I carefully weighed on my accurate letter scales. They came to just under a kilogram, so I walked with the parcel containing them to the post office about 40 minutes away. But when I placed the parcel on the post office scales it weighed just over a kilogram. It was entirely my fault as I'd weighed the presents before wrapping them. So, I cheerily said, 'Oh dear, when I weighed them at home they were just under a kilogram,' to which the person behind the counter replied, 'Well, that's why your cakes are never a success!'

His assumption – which had nothing to do with the issue at hand – unsettled me so that I was unable to explain that I'd weighed the contents unwrapped. Things went downhill from there. My suggestion that I open the parcel and take something out was roundly rejected. (I could have bought some Sellotape and stuck it together again!) I made other suggestions, which were also rejected. Then a customs form was shoved across the counter and I was told to fill it in, which I can't do without help. I left in tears and came home, still carrying the parcel.

As I arrived back at the village I met a rather agitated lady standing outside our village shop holding half a cup of milk. She told me she had hoped to move to a place where there was a shop, but she had become very distressed, as she'd found out that she couldn't buy any milk here as there was no shop and the milk in the cup was all she had. I told her she was right, 'You can't buy any milk right now, because the shop is closed at present,' but added that, 'The shop does open again at nine o'clock tomorrow morning.' I reassured her that she had enough milk for at least two cups of tea which would last her until then, and soon she was settled and happy again. I did wonder what the person behind the post office counter would have said to her!

A little kindness can make an enormous difference to the person on the receiving end. One day my intercom rang to inform me a food delivery had arrived. I assured the person it couldn't be mine as I had received it yesterday – there must be a mistake. The delivery man was exceptional: he alerted the office staff, who let him in through the main doors, and he brought it all up to my flat on the first floor. On further rejection by myself he asked me politely, as he was there, if I would just check my fridge to see if I had enough milk . . . Whoops, it was almost empty! I apologized and explained that I had dementia. He smiled and said his mum also had dementia and frequently sent away deliveries as she had forgotten she'd ordered them. I sent the firm an email to thank them for his persistence.

It's good to be able to tell retailers when they are doing a good job. But if on the other hand they are not, it can be an opportunity to bring this to their attention so that they can put it right. I once took a lot of coins in to my bank from the sales at a conference of my teaching DVDs and USB sticks. I wasn't able to count them and handed them over at the counter in various bags. There were three women behind the screens, and no other customers in the building. But they refused to count the coins for me, and told me to fill in a form once I had counted them myself. I had no idea which form and where to find it, and 'over there' was not helpful. It was only when I sat and cried that one of the staff said she wasn't allowed to add them up as she might add them up incorrectly. 'Well,' I said through my tears, 'I would certainly add them up incorrectly, so I would be none the wiser!' And I left. But to do something positive with that experience, I then got involved in another bank's dementia awareness training.

Soon after I arrived in the village I visited the local library. I was having difficulty reading books and had almost given up, but I chose some books in large print written for people with learning disabilities. I took six of them up to the counter and presented my bus pass. The staff just stood and laughed at me. I couldn't understand why, as in Southampton we could use our bus passes at the library and leisure facilities. Also, might the fact that the books were for people with learning disabilities have given them a clue that I needed help? I vowed never to go back there again, but my son insisted that I did, so we went; he watched proceedings from a distance. I was given a form to complete and I filled it in with my old Southampton address and a completely wrong date of birth. However, the lady on duty that day asked me very gently if perhaps I would like some help to fill in the form . . . such a difference!

Using buses can be another trial. One day I got on the wrong bus and only realized when it turned right instead of left at a crossroads. The driver just shouted at me, although I'd told him when I got on where I wanted to go. Another driver was very abrupt when I forgot how to use my bus pass, and yet another told me to get off the bus as it wasn't yet 9.30 in the morning – the time that concessionary bus passes start – though it was half past nine by my watch, and the bus was almost empty. I ended up in tears at the roadside.

Because of these experiences my son and I made a laminated card for me to show the driver when I got on, or to present at the bank or library, or to the appropriate person in similar situations anywhere, before saying anything. But whether or not someone has dementia, how can those uncaring attitudes be justified?

The Alzheimer's Society's Dementia Friendly Communities initiative has done sterling work in educating people about dementia and inspiring them to create dementia-friendly communities. Large retailers like Marks & Spencer and Tesco and high street banks have also invested in training their staff. But it can take a while for this to filter through to everyone.

The enabling power of love

Professor Kitwood (1997) said that when it comes to helping someone with dementia, 'there is only one all-encompassing need – for love'. He put love at the centre of a compass that includes attachment, comfort, sense of identity, occupation and inclusion. Jesus also put love at the centre of our lives when He said, '"You shall love the Lord your God with all your heart and with all your soul and with all your mind and with all your strength . . ." The second is this: "You shall love your neighbour as yourself." There is no other commandment greater than these' (Mark 12.30–31, esv). There are many ways, large and small, of showing love to someone with dementia. I've already touched on some of them here: visiting and bringing 'good feelings', bringing laughter (with us, not at us), listening, helping to put things right, being patient, looking for the emotion behind the words, and helping to avoid sensory overload.

And to those of us to whom God is important, tell us of God's unconditional love, acceptance and forgiveness. We can forget even the basic Christian truths, so remind us of them. When visiting a frightened woman with advanced dementia, I take a tear-off sheet from a daily Bible verse calendar. She sits holding it with a smile on her face. Enabling us to remember God's truth can bring us joy. When we are overwhelmed by not knowing who people are, when I'm getting lost, when I can't find a place, when my hallucinations of animals or dangerous situations occur, when people are rude or unhelpful, this is what I remember:

> There will be a highway called the Holy Road. No one rude or rebellious is permitted on this road. It's for God's people exclusively – impossible to get lost on this road . . . No lions on this road, no dangerous wild animals – Nothing and no one dangerous or threatening.
>
> Only the redeemed will walk on it . . . They'll sing as they make

their way home to Zion, unfading halos of joy encircling their heads,
Welcomed home with gifts of joy and gladness as all sorrows and
sighs scurry into the night. (Isaiah 35.8–10, *THE MESSAGE*)

Indeed, what joy! No one rude is allowed on this road, and
there will be nothing dangerous or threatening. It's a high-
way I'm looking forward to taking and, even as I consider it,
I wonder if there will be bright red poppies growing along the
wayside.

7

A full life,
even with exploding bananas

Writing notes for a talk I was to give recently, I was reminded of a frightening event in 2001, the year I went back to Mseleni Hospital for the second time. The first time I returned, in 1971, I found myself at times the only doctor there, feeling the weight of the responsibility. It was something I had told God I would never do! But we must be careful not to tell God things we could never do, as He has ways of showing us that we can – that His grace is sufficient, whatever our circumstances (2 Corinthians 12.9).

When I went back in 2001 the hospital was being staffed by eight to ten doctors. We would spend some of our off-duty time relaxing on the beach. It was a beautiful beach, wide and unspoiled. We were there one day when suddenly, without warning, the sea water rushed in and the beach was totally submerged. It was completely unexpected, and some of our party were almost swept away. We were very glad that the keys had been left in the Land Rover further up the beach, because we lost everything else that we'd taken with us that day. We were so thankful that the two people who'd been in real difficulty in the water hadn't drowned.

It's almost a parable of how our plans can all be swept away in a moment. When this happens, people can feel that their lives have come to an end. I'm sure that's how Jonah felt when he found himself inside the massive fish. It's a good picture of how people can feel; trapped and submerged by their problems, surrounded by darkness and with no way out. But Jonah's life didn't end inside the big fish. It spat him out on to a beach and he quickly realized that he still had an important job to do. He still had a relationship with God, and could both hear from Him and talk to Him. Proverbs 19.21 says, 'Many are the plans in a person's heart, but it is the LORD's purpose that prevails' (NIV).

God's purpose is not for us to have the difficulty, but for Him to show His love to us and to others, enabling us to experience Him in a new and deeper way. I feel I know God far better now than I did before I had dementia. A diagnosis of dementia doesn't mean that life has come to an end. The fact that I am writing this book ten years after being diagnosed witnesses to that.

However, like any other illness, as dementia progresses people need more and more support from others. When diagnosed with young-onset dementia people are relatively youthful (as the name implies) and there can be more capacity at that stage to reorder life and put in place support structures than when you are older. People in their eighties and nineties tend to have fewer social and family contacts, and charities such as Age UK show that the lack of social care funding means that many have very little, if any, support. With the largest generation of older people in history, this is a growing challenge for all concerned, including government, social services, families, and especially individuals with dementia themselves.

I've been blessed by being surrounded by marvellous people all my life. I knew Stanley loved me dearly, but I didn't expect him or any other family member to care for me when I became permanently 'adrift', which is one of the reasons he and I moved to the village. My siblings are supportive, and have had me to stay with them at various times or have helped me in other ways.

The pillars of my support base are my adult children and their spouses. David runs my website and makes my videos. Paul has edited articles I've written, as has Alison; and Alison's husband Andy dealt with my medication until they moved overseas. They've all accompanied me to conferences. Although one lives in London and the others live overseas, thanks to technology, we talk face-to-face frequently over Skype. This was a lifesaver on one occasion, when David connected with me from Ukraine and could see that there was something wrong with me. He asked a few questions, rang off, and within minutes a carer appeared. She arranged for me to be taken to my GP, who said I needed to be 'blue-lighted' by ambulance to hospital. It helps too that, if necessary, David and Paul can be here within a few hours. After the 'blue-light' incident David got on the next available plane and was at the hospital the next day.

Living with dementia calls for planning

All my life I've been an early riser, and I usually wake at 6 a.m. and listen to my daily Bible reading for half an hour. This comes by DAB (Daily Audio Bible), and if I'm not sleeping well I'll listen to it during the night as well. The DAB programme goes through the Bible in a year, which is wonderful for me because I can't remember what I heard yesterday. Night-times can be like Psalm 63.6–7, which says, 'On my bed I remember you . . . I sing in the shadow of your wings' (NIV).

Night-time can be difficult for people with dementia. Mine are usually disturbed and can even be frightening or distressing. Because of the dementia, I'm never sure what actually happens during the night. Hallucinations are as real at night as they are during the day, though smells are no worse, fortunately. Sometimes an hallucination can be so out of context that it's obvious, such as the time an ambulance seemed to be backing into my bedroom. There's no way an ambulance could have been driven up the stairs, so I just laughed. The doorbell sounding, or the telephone ringing, are minor inconveniences as long as I realize soon enough not to waste time hunting for the source. If I have remembered to lock my front door I know that the people I see are not real, but I feel that I can never be absolutely sure until I try the front door in the morning. I'm still puzzling over the mystery of how, one morning, I woke with a glorious black eye, with my nightdress on the bathroom floor while I was wearing something different.

Once out of bed in the morning it's into the bathroom, and if I'm due to wash my hair the shampoo will be on the floor in the shower. Only shower gel is kept by the shower head. In the past I've used various other liquids by mistake, so they are now all kept elsewhere. My toothbrush and toothpaste are the first thing I see, alongside my hand basin – no other tubes are kept there.

I get dressed from the pile of clothes on the floor in the order they are laid out. Appearing in public with one's petticoat (or anything else) on top of one's dress is not a good idea! Having my clothes in a pile in the order in which they are to be put on helps avoid this, and I make sure they are placed that way the night before.

The next step then is to press the 'OK' button on my phone set on the way to the kitchen. Sometimes I don't do this, because I've forgotten to leave my cardboard reminder notice in the right place, but if I don't press the button I'm automatically phoned at 8.40 a.m. to ask if I am all right. If I go out without having done these checks the staff will be concerned and will come looking for me.

I make a cup of tea and when I take the milk out of the fridge I see my rainbow medication box telling me which day it is. I remove it, take my morning medication and place it on my tea caddy to remind me to take later doses. For breakfast I have cereal and yoghurt, and if all has gone well, everything is completed before my alarm goes off to remind me to take my medication and have breakfast. Staff here will also check this.

A tech-savvy generation

After breakfast I open my laptop and look at my digital calendar to see what I'm meant to be doing today. It tells me everything: whether I'm due to go to the gym, go swimming, run my memory groups, help with outside community groups involved with disabled people, change my bed linen, defrost the freezer or send someone a birthday card – any number of things. It also tells me if I am expecting visitors. This is important because, if I am not expecting them, I might not know who people are when they arrive. My calendar is colour coded so I can easily view all my talks and lectures across the month, as well as my family's activities, or events that are taking place in my village. Thank God for computers! I used to have a PC but found it a struggle, so my son David persuaded me to change to a Mac. It is perfect for me: it links to my iPad and my son can deal with things from Ukraine. We both benefit from the Internet-connected world.

A lack of technological awareness was something I found very frustrating shortly after receiving my diagnosis, when Stanley and I were looking at possible future residential facilities. We looked all around the country and found brand new buildings with old furniture and ancient click-clack typewriters. At one place I asked if they had Wi-Fi. 'What's that?' asked the manager. 'Is it a kind of game?' (She may have been thinking of the Wii!) In contrast, the St Monica's Trust, who run my village, are excellent and are always seeking to improve.

There was almost nothing provided for those with young-onset dementia. Things have changed over the last ten years, because many of us around the world have been making our voices heard. Kate Swaffer and Richard Taylor's organization, Dementia Alliance International, has made great progress providing a 'unified voice of strength, advocacy and support' for people diagnosed with dementia. It also has online support groups and webinars (seminars conducted over the internet). Dementia Mentors, set up by Gary Le Blanc, is another excellent online resource for people with dementia, holding online dementia chat groups (dementia cafés) and offering individual, one-on-one mentoring.

We have grown up in a computer-savvy generation and we retain those skills. I can remember going to the launch of an iPad test for dementia that I'd been involved with. It had been developed by Cambridge Cognition, and was suitable for all abilities and all ethnic backgrounds. I was sitting next to a famous newspaper computer software reporter who laughed at me for suggesting that there was any future in such developments. (I still have his name!)

I spend an hour looking at or deleting emails – I'm quite ruthless, as otherwise I get overwhelmed, since I receive about 80 a day. I learned as a doctor only to read anything once and deal with it straight away; it's a habit that still stands me in good stead. I am at my best in the morning, so I often write important emails then, and I try to never leave more than ten emails in my inbox to deal with later. Mornings are also the best time for dealing with my internet bank. The bank is aware of my diagnosis and can alert my eldest son if there are concerns. The joy of my Mac is that it stores my passwords and completes forms with my details automatically.

I find shops almost impossible to deal with and confine myself to a very short list of internet shopping outlets. My daughter and daughter-in-law have set up a system for me, a 'favourites' list to choose from, which enables me to order household items on the internet once every two weeks.

There was a time when I could give a lecture without notes, but now I write out every word I am planning to say, because I can't remember if I have said something earlier. I also know how many words I can have in my notes to ensure I don't go over the allocated time. Again, I prepare lectures earlier in the day. I never give exactly the same talk twice, partly because I am always learning something new and partly because there may be someone in the audience who has heard it before!

One day I started my lecture by saying I was going to show a two-minute video to give an idea of how living with dementia felt from the inside. (It wasn't a video from my website.) I was having difficulty getting it to play, when a loud voice from the front said, 'Don't bother – I've seen it three times already!' That was the only time anything like this ever happened. I replied, 'No you haven't! This is a new one and no one has seen it yet!'

I have two similar versions of this video. One has music and written words accompanying still photographs, which I was told was not acceptable as blind people could not benefit from it. So we made one with music and spoken words and was told that was not acceptable either, as deaf people were unable to benefit from it. Nowadays, when I plan to use the video, I send my notes to the conference organizers beforehand, so they can decide which version will suit their anticipated audience.

In the morning I might also talk to other people with dementia around the world on Zoom, a video conferencing program for online meetings that enables up to 25 people to talk together. Then I might go to the gym, go swimming, prepare the residents' coffee morning, run my Japanese Memory Groups or prepare materials for them.

There was a time when I used to forget to eat or drink and lost a lot of weight, so my family has arranged for a hot meal to be brought to me three times a week. I leave all my crockery in the bowl in the sink and only wash up once a day, so I know what I have eaten and how many cups of tea or glasses of water or apple juice I have had. The restaurant here is brilliant and when I get muddled as to which day it is they always look after me, and sort things out graciously.

If I'm having a bad day I might forget how to do things, as the ability to sequence goes. The local Alzheimer's Society introduced me to an inspired young man called Will Britton, who was working on QR codes (a sort of barcode) to bring up short videos on personal iPads to give reminders to people with learning disabilities or dementia. These range from making a cup of tea, using the microwave and changing quilt covers, to what to take when you leave home – for example, keys, money and bus pass.

On a good day I might do some simple cooking. I have a single, double-sided laminated sheet with my 'best personal recipes' from over the years, such as scones, biscuits, cakes, jam and marmalade. Once I made some rock buns to welcome my son David, but he had to put them all in the bin because I'd forgotten the sugar. On another occasion I used salt instead of sugar. But he knows how to treat me: he insists, 'You can't hide behind your dementia, Mum, find a way to do it properly!' When I ruined lemon curd by forgetting to include the eggs, I learned that I have to get out all the ingredients beforehand and lay them out in a line and put everything else away before I begin.

Exploding bananas

One one occasion, not putting things away almost resulted in disaster. The internet delivery man had very kindly put everything in the kitchen for me, but had left some items on the cooker hob. Normally, I just put the items away. This time, though, I didn't. I just moved enough aside, turned on the hob and put on a saucepan – but turned on the wrong burner. Then I turned all four burners on full, with the plastic bags of shopping still on top. I could see the red hobs, and I could see the plastic melting, and the cardboard turning into carbon – I could see everything happening, but I didn't realize its significance. And then I could smell it, the burning and the scorching, but I just thought 'hallucination!' It was only when the bananas exploded – when the third sense, hearing, came in – that I realized what was happening. Even though I could see it and smell it, it didn't mean anything to me.

Since then I've been very careful when cooking, always making sure the hob is clear. But I have to be equally careful about remembering what I'm doing if there is an interruption. On one occasion the doorbell went, and I left the kitchen to answer it and forgot that I was cooking. I came back into the sitting room and sat down, and got on with some knitting.

After a while I noticed the smell of supper cooking, and thought how good it was, and wondered if it was coming from the people downstairs. It didn't enter my head that it was my supper – often I can't remember whether or not I have eaten anyway. I thought, 'Oh well, maybe it's an hallucination.' A little bit later, the 'supper' began to smell a bit overcooked, and later still it began to smell a bit burnt, and I thought, 'Well, it's definitely an hallucination, you can stop worrying about it now.'

Of course, it got worse and worse. At one stage I went into

the dining room to check my emails, and still didn't think of looking in the kitchen. Eventually it got really bad, so I thought, 'Well, I'm obviously suffering from bad hallucinations today. I'll go and make myself a cup of tea.' I went into the kitchen and – oh dear!

It's a terrible fire risk, so when I start cooking I put a timer around my neck, set for, say, half an hour. Then, should I get distracted from what I'm doing, the timer will go off and remind me to go into the kitchen to have a look. I need to have systems and precautions in place so that I can continue to live independently.

Although I do all that I can, I'm comforted in knowing that God is in charge of my life. His attention to detail never fails to amaze me – even, on one occasion, down to the precise number of pennies! I mentioned it in my leaving talk as a GP. When Stanley was made redundant all our outgoings had to be covered by my earnings. In those days GPs' salaries were paid out of the monies left after all the practice's bills had been covered, including the mortgage, staff salaries, utility bills, medical dressings and drugs and so on. One day I said to our practice manager that I'd worked out how much I needed that month, right down to the pennies, and I told her what the amount was – pounds, shillings and pence. She said, 'How many did you say?' I repeated the pounds, but she said again, 'No, the pennies!' Then she handed me the salary cheque that had been made out earlier – and it was the exact amount I'd said, down to the pennies!

* * *

In the afternoon I will visit people in their flats, and others in the care home. I especially like to visit people that others don't bother with. It's a blessing to me, as I love people, but it can be draining. Sometimes, when my energy has run out, I will shut my door and do nothing.

Early in the evening I get out my dress for the next day. I don't wear clothes with zips or buttons as they can be done up incorrectly or left undone. My daughter made the brilliant discovery of a reversible dress, which she bought me, which I still find rather wonderful. How enterprising of companies to make a range of reversible clothing for people with dementia! There are already so many helpful, innovative products, such as brightly coloured tablecloths which contrast with white crockery, digital day and date clocks, simple music players where you just have to lift the lid, and an extra simple mobile phone that also acts as a GPS tracker should the person get lost. There are even insoles for shoes that contain GPS trackers. The Alzheimer's Society sells many different items, as does a brilliant organization called Unforgettable.

Before I go to bed I check my computer for emails and read instructions for the next day, especially those that tell me if I need to leave anything on the floor, or in the hall, where I will walk over it and so be sure to notice it – this works well for me.

Staying away from home

For people with dementia, staying away from home can be another challenge. I need confidence that if I become confused, someone will know how to help me. Once I tried to sleep in a cupboard thinking the metal storage shelves were my bed: I was with my son in Ukraine at the time and we had a good laugh about it. If I am speaking at a conference with an early morning start I will usually stay somewhere nearby the night before. I almost always stay in a Premier Inn as they are all almost identical, and hence familiar and predictable. It helps, too, that the staff are friendly and helpful.

From Richard Taylor, the author of *Dementia from the Inside Out*, I learned the therapeutic benefit of writing about things in order to help cope with them, so I've recorded many of these in my blog. I am so grateful for the empathy of others with dementia, and as you can see, I'm equally thankful for the love and support of my family.

Supporting families

Many times, I've observed the depth of empathy and the extraordinary love and patience that family members show to those living with dementia (or other disabilities). I see, too, their *preparedness*; willingness is not a strong enough word to describe the motivation to go not just the second, but the third mile. Sadly, this is not universal, and I've noticed some who are impatient or unwilling to help, or who just withdraw. I'm aware that they themselves have needs and feelings, and many families will have strains and fractures long before dementia appears. In *Dementia Reconsidered* Tom Kitwood includes chapters about the perceptions and emotions of families and caregivers, and says that negative emotions must be left outside the door, as far as possible, before spending time with someone with dementia.

There sometimes comes a time when residential care is best for the person with dementia, and his or her family. In a care home there are teams of staff who have been trained to give the best care, and who support one another. They get time off – and importantly, they get a night's good sleep! Relieved of the stress of caring 24 hours a day, families can develop richer relationships with those with dementia. And people often improve in a care home. They are relieved of the responsibilities they felt in their own home; that load is lifted from them. An example is Douglas, who went into residential care for two weeks' respite when his son and daughter-in-law acted on their doctor's advice and took a holiday. Douglas enjoyed the company of others in the home and the activities and, more importantly, felt it lifted an increasingly heavy burden of care from his family's shoulders. He asked their pastor to explain to his son that he was happy in the home, he felt safe, and he had company.

So, it isn't because the care their family has been giving isn't good enough: it's no reflection on the way they have looked after the person before. I feel very strongly about this. The wife of someone I knew had dementia and he cared for her for far longer than he should have done, because he'd promised she would never have to go into residential care. But when he fell and broke his hip and hurt a shoulder there was no way he could care for her, so he had to find a place for her in a care home. Then, when he went to church on Sunday, people said, 'How could you do that?' The third time someone said that to him, he tried to kill himself. We need to affirm people when they do things that they might not want to do, not blame them. Feelings of guilt are corrosive and destructive.

Guilt weighs us down, and we often experience it because we are not seeing things as we ought. How did Jesus feel about Judas? Jesus had chosen him, and appointed him as one of His disciples, so when it became clear that Judas was a thief, did Jesus feel guilty? It must have been tough for Jesus, and I wonder if sometimes that was part of the pain He felt in the Garden. Did He feel that He'd failed with Judas? Did He feel that He'd failed when the disciples didn't understand some of the things He taught; that they hadn't grasped the significance of what He told them about His death and resurrection? We are not responsible for the consequences of our obedience to God, and Jesus always did what pleased His Father. There is no evidence that Jesus ever had feelings of guilt, or that He felt a failure.

When Jesus wept outside the tomb of Lazarus, He wasn't weeping for Lazarus, because He knew that he was going to come back to life again. He cared deeply for Lazarus and his sisters. When Lazarus fell ill, and they sent for Him, He took a long time to arrive. He was met by Mary, who was crying and blaming Him for not coming sooner. The Scriptures say that Jesus was deeply moved in spirit, and troubled. The word 'troubled' means agitated, confused, fearful, falling apart; heading for a meltdown. So, what did Jesus do? It's the shortest verse in the Bible – He wept. Jesus knew beforehand that the incident was for God's glory. He'd said, 'This sickness will not end in death. No, it is for God's glory so that God's Son may be glorified through it' (John 11.4, NIV). In delaying His arrival He was obeying His Father, and although deeply moved and upset, He was content to leave the consequences to God.

* * *

In Matthew 7.12 Jesus says, 'So in everything, do to others what you would have them do to you, for this sums up the Law and the Prophets' (NIV). This principle is central to the care of people with dementia. Think how you would like people to be towards you, if you had dementia. Don't disable us – *enable us*, with understanding and kindness. Be patient if we seem slow, and understand when we are time travelling.

8

Kintsukuroi

This has been my story of how I learned to live well with dementia, and the simple principles I discovered that can dramatically alter the lives of everyone affected by the condition, whether they have been diagnosed with it, or are caring for someone, or simply living in a society where so many people are affected. If these principles were understood and adopted by everyone the whole of society would benefit, not just people with dementia. Tom Kitwood has written, in *Dementia Reconsidered* (1997), that 'all events in human interaction, great and small, have their counterpart at a neurological level', and that 'because of their life experience and learning, individuals may vary considerably in the extent to which they are able to withstand processes in the brain that destroy synapses, and hence in their resistance to dementia'.

The principles that I've learned are mentioned in Chapter 5. Let me remind you of them.

1 *There is always a reason* why a person is behaving in a particular way .
2 *When facts are forgotten, feelings remain.*
3 *Familiar patterns of behaviour continue.*

Knowing these principles can help explain puzzling behaviour and improve communications. In his book *Contented Dementia* (2010), psychologist Oliver James describes how a care home resident was found in the kitchen, holding a knife, by the cook when she went on duty. She pushed the emergency button and the resident was taken to the mental ward of a local hospital and given antipsychotic drugs. Yet analysis of the situation showed that he had been a chef, and when the incident occurred he had been time travelling, thinking he was going to work.

If the cook had known about the resident's background she would have known that it was a familiar pattern of behaviour for him. Countless times in his life he had gone into a big kitchen to work, and would naturally pick up a knife. So clearly, it helps to know as much as possible about the person. On the whole, family members know each other well, but nursing and care homes have to acquire the information from relatives. Living in the village and getting to know people, I'm learning a lot about their histories and they have come to know something of mine!

Remember, too, that a person's meltdown, or their responsive behaviour, is the result of fear, sensory overload or other environmental triggers, as outlined in Chapter 5. Identifying and avoiding these triggers helps to keep the person on an even keel. Dr Graham Stokes, Director of Dementia Care at BUPA, the healthcare provider with residential homes in the UK, has described how individuals' past life experiences are responsible for their reactions (Stokes, 2010). For example, the lady who would scream non-stop when in the home's lounge was found to have a phobia about cats; not knowing this, carers would position her wheelchair so she could look out of the window – but on the windowsill was a large statuette of a cat.

Sometimes triggers are less obvious: a carer in a residential home needed to help a lady with dementia, whom she knew quite well, but when she knocked on her door and entered her room the resident shouted at her to get out and leave her alone. The carer went out, waited a moment or two and took off her cardigan before going back in. The resident beamed at her and said, 'Oh it's you! I know that you love me, but I didn't like that other girl.' Getting on with the job in hand, the carer replied with a smile, 'I don't like her myself, sometimes!' She couldn't remember if she'd worn that particular cardigan before, but assumed that the resident's visual perception might have had something to do with her behaviour that day (Morse, 2010).

These principles have been illustrated through each chapter. Perhaps one of the most important requirements for helping people with dementia is empathy, the ability to understand and share the feelings of another. It's not the same as sympathy, which is feeling sorrow or compassion, or even pity for another's misfortune. Empathy is more to do with putting oneself in the other person's shoes. There was little empathy from the man behind the counter at the post office when I'd misjudged the weight of my parcel, whereas the lady behind the counter at the library who helped me complete the membership form showed a great deal of it.

Another example is a local taxi firm who know exactly how to treat me. I sit in the back of the car and sometimes like to chat; at other times I say that I would rather travel quietly. The driver never gets flustered and is utterly reliable. I'm able to travel alone with him, and when we arrive at our destination, sometimes after several hours, he'll announce that he is going in to find 'the facilities', so I ask if I can tag along. He waits for me and then makes sure I end up in the right place with the right people. I often think that finding 'the facilities' is just for my benefit, but in a way that causes no embarrassment.

In contrast, I once travelled with a taxi driver who got in such a state because some roads were closed, and he had another fare to collect, that I asked to be let out near the destination and said I would walk. Unfortunately, it wasn't as easy as I thought; even though I had a map of my destination I needed to ask several people to help. When I eventually arrived, the meeting had started and I was in tears – not a good beginning! (I am sometimes reminded of this by others who were there, but only in a friendly, supportive way.)

One of the best examples of empathy I've experienced happened during a visit to one of my favourite places. Stanley and I both enjoyed gardens, and the beautiful Bishop Palace Gardens were the nearest to us at Sandford. We loved it so much we became founder life members of the place. Sadly, Stanley died before we could enjoy our membership, so I arranged to have a bench placed overlooking the water from the wells, with the cathedral in the background. It is really the best place in the gardens and a very peaceful spot. I love being there, so I was delighted when Rosie Martin, the chief executive, invited me to visit to see this year's exceptional tulips. Rosie met me off the bus, and when I didn't spot her she called out my name and waved her identification label and smiled. Before we met anyone, she reminded me of when I had last seen them, and how they had helped me, so I was able to thank them. Thoughtfulness like this is so refreshing, and doubled the blessing of being there.

* * *

In a relatively short time recently there have been two different media reports that illustrate the difference that empathy, or the lack of it, makes to the well-being of people with dementia. In an article with the headline, 'Rementia: is it possible to reverse the symptoms of early-stage dementia?' occupational therapist Jackie Pool, Head of Memory at Sunrise Senior Living, is advocating an individualized programme of occupational therapy for people with dementia that can maintain their current abilities, and help restore lost functions by enabling the creation of new links between neurons in place of those that have been damaged. Patterns can continue and skills can be reused, even in different ways.

When she first worked as an occupational therapy assistant in the 1980s Ms Pool had been shocked by the treatment of people with dementia, who had simply been given up on. Now, she says, the culture has changed, and we know that how we treat people with dementia is crucial to their well-being. There are many other individualized programmes of care up and down the country, and here in the village we have a marvellous dementia activities organizer (Wayne) who has made a tremendous difference. But there is still so much more to be done.

The second account is of a government-funded study of how patients with dementia are treated in some NHS hospitals. Researchers found that staff in five major hospitals were confining patients with dementia to their beds by raising the side-rails, tucking bedsheets tightly around them, putting their walking frames out of reach or sedating them with drugs. When patients became unhappy and resistant to treatment, staff assumed it was because of their dementia. The patients' group were seen as difficult to handle and very needy, and there was a strong sense that staff resented them being there. The report said that these tactics resulted in the 'dehumanization' of patients and a worsening of their already poor health. Staff lacked skills training, and a shortage of nurses meant they didn't have the time to talk to patients about their lives or look at old photographs with them to give them mental stimulus. The report only covered five hospitals, and it certainly wasn't my experience when I was in an acute medical ward in 2016, in the Bristol Royal Infirmary. The staff there were brilliant, as I mentioned in Chapter 5.

* * *

The use of language about people with dementia also makes a great difference, and I'm sure that moderating the way we describe dementia has played a part in reducing stigma over the last ten years. Language is important, because it influences and defines perceptions. Many of the negative connotations attached to dementia relate to the words that are used, and the result, for many, is a lack of hope. Many conditions force us to negotiate dreadful paths, such as cancer, strokes, multiple sclerosis – all kinds of disabilities – but we don't use the same language about them. So rather than referring to a 'dementia sufferer', which denotes the person as a victim, why not use the term 'person with dementia' or 'person living with dementia'? There are times, of course, when we do suffer, and so do those around us, but that does not define who we are.

An example of good language use is the Canadian term 'responsive behaviour', indicating that there is a reason for an individual's behaviour. Other words that convey meaning are 'rementia'; 'requesting', which can prevent confrontation, instead of 'insisting'; 'reconsider' when things are not going well; and 'rephrase' your sentence or 'redirect' rather than shouting when there is not an immediate response. Reassure and reinforce what is good and helpful. And a reminder – please don't ask, 'Do you remember . . .?' when you first meet us as it can make us freeze inside and prevent us from responding easily. But if you say, 'I remember when . . .' that can carry us along, and we can join in.

Enabling speech

I have found there are five main ways of helping those in the later stages of dementia to talk, when others assume they no longer can – it is such a joy! The key words here are music, singing, laughter, and parallel and convergent speech.

Music

Access to music is easy nowadays, using smartphones or iPads or other tablets. They are light and portable and can hold so much. As neurologist Oliver Sacks remarked in the YouTube video I referred to earlier, music has a quickening effect on the brain. You'll remember that the nursing home in the YouTube video matched the music to the residents' likes and experiences.

Singing

I have found that singing ties up loose ends, and as with the lady who kept repeating that 'the peas are green on Saturday', it can have a releasing effect, like moving on a stuck record.

Laughter

Laughter too has a releasing effect. I was laughing with a lady with advanced dementia recently; she normally says very little, but she suddenly started telling me stories about her childhood that I hadn't heard before. Among other things, laughter reduces stress and tension.

Paralleling

Talk about something and see if the person will join in. It involves looking for a topic of interest, a hook that will draw the person in, so he or she will continue the conversation along with you.

Converging

This is where you join in with whatever the person is talking about, even if the person isn't making sense. Note the emotional pattern of the conversation, and reflect back the emotion using any recognized words. It's so rewarding when the person begins to talk sense.

Visual communications

The Dementia Friendly Communities initiative has helped a great deal in practical ways, such as better understanding; good street lighting, road signage, and so on. I wish they would look at public toilets in hotels, restaurants, motorway service stations . . . wherever they are. They are a nightmare! I need a clearly signposted exit trail. I have spent untold time trying to find the way out, when all doorways look the same, and mirrors compound the problem. Then how to lock the toilet door is often a mystery, and unlocking it even more so. I've been involved with many people with dementia, helping them, in such situations. Then, how do I turn on these taps, or get the soap out of the dispenser, and what's the hand drying procedure here? Yet these problems could be solved quite easily by pictures and diagrams. Small print instructions are no help at all.

*　*　*

In my talks, I like to sum up the ways to stay well and to help others stay well with an acronym – SLEDGE. When I mentioned this recently someone laughed and said, 'Oh, at the top of the slippery slope!' But this is not the case at all – sledges can be fun, and are also used on level ground. Think of sledges used across ice, for example. SLEDGE stands for Laughter, Exercise, Diet and coGnitive stimulation, all within the context of Social Engagement.

The value of social engagement, another way of saying spending time with other people, is supported by increasing scientific evidence. A Finnish study called FINGER (Kivipelto, 2013), involving 1,260 older people in a two-year study that included diet, exercise, cognitive training and vascular risk monitoring (and treatment if necessary), found this 'multi-domain' approach could improve or maintain cognitive functioning in at-risk elderly people.

In studies of ageing, scientists have discovered regions in the world where people live exceptionally long, healthy lives. These regions are called 'Blue Zones', and researchers have found that the primary reason for longevity is the social connections of individuals who live there. Psychologist Susan Pinker, in a TED talk, refers to research showing that quite simple interactions, such as making eye contact with another person, and shaking hands, releases beneficial hormones. (To watch the talk, Google 'The secret to living longer', Susan Pinker.)

Robin Dunbar, Professor of Experimental Psychology at Oxford University, says the same. At a Times Scientific seminar in Cheltenham in 2015 he said that it is our relationships that have the strongest impact on survival, even with patients who have had heart attacks. Yet, 'despite these findings, the importance of social networks has been ignored completely by the medical profession,' he added.

People with dementia benefit greatly from social interaction. They can and should still lead active lives, taking exercise and meeting regularly with groups. The Alzheimer's Society has many suggestions on its website, including singing groups, arts and crafts such as painting or knitting, visiting places of interest such as botanical gardens, and dementia cafés. Although the focus in Professor Kawashima's work was on cognitive stimulation, social interaction played a large part, and it is the same with my JMGs here in the village.

Some authorities have purchased robots to help in residential care homes. These can include robotic pets, which have been found to be quite popular, although a care home manager warns against letting the batteries run out as residents with dementia may assume the pet has died. Robots might have a useful place for people living alone as they can alert others to falls and unusual behaviour. However, most of all, people need people. Giving people with dementia your time, your energy, your love can be costly, but the rewards are great. Seeing someone relax, smile and communicate is worth the effort.

Reading Proverbs 5.21 reminded me of how detailed is God's care of us. It says, 'For your ways are in full view of the LORD, and he examines all your paths' (NIV). I had this image of God on His hands and knees examining my paths, looking for the potholes and the jagged stones. This is amazing – that God, the Creator of the universe, examines all our paths. He knows exactly what hazards lie ahead, because He has examined our paths. People think God doesn't care, but He is there with us, watching over us.

Broken vessels more precious than before

Kintsukuroi is the Japanese art of repairing broken pottery with costly gold or silver, making it more beautiful and of greater worth than before. My African pot that arrived in a hundred pieces, and which I so carefully put back together, is more precious to me now because of the time and care I invested in it. But it's not just the time spent with Kintsukuroi; the value comes from the precious elements that are gluing it together.

The art of Kintsukuroi is a wonderful picture to me of how God has poured his love and grace into my life to hold it together, making it more beautiful and giving it greater value. It is also a picture of how we can all pour love and care and acceptance into the lives of those around us, making them more beautiful. No matter how cracked or broken their lives, we can show they are of immense value.

Bibliography and further reading

Alzheimer's Research UK, dementia statistics, diagnoses in the UK, at: <www.dementiastatistics.org/statistics/diagnoses-in-the-uk>.

Bute, J. (2011) 'A Patient's Journey: Dementia with cardiac problems', *British Medical Journal*, 343:d4278.

Dementia Alliance International, <www.dementiaallianceinternational.org>.

Dementia Mentors, <www.dementiamentors.org>.

Flint, A. J. (2016) in L. B. E. Cowman, *Streams in the Desert Morning and Evening: 365 devotions.* London: Zondervan.

James, O. (2010) *Contented Dementia.* London: Vermilion.

Kawashima, R. (2013) 'Mental exercises for cognitive function: Clinical evidence', *Journal of Preventive Medicine and Public Health*, January, 46 (Supplement 1): S22–S27. (Available online at: <www.ncbi.nlm.nih.gov/pmc/articles/PMC3567314>.)

Kitwood, T. (1997) *Dementia Reconsidered.* Milton Keynes: Open University Press.

Kivipelto, M., et al. (2013) 'The Finnish geriatric study to prevent cognitive impairment and disability (FINGER): Study design and progress', *Alzheimer's and Dementia*, November, 9(6): 657–65. (Available online at: <www.ncbi.nlm.nih.gov/pubmed/23332672>.)

Matthews, F. E., et al. (2016) 'A two decade comparison of incidence of dementia in individuals aged 65 years and older from three geographical areas of England: Results of the Cognitive Function Ageing Study I and II', *Nature Communications*, 19 April, DOI: 10.1038/ncomms11398. (Available online at: <www.cam.ac.uk/research/news/new-cases-of-dementia-in-the-uk-fall-by-20-over-two-decades>.)

Morse, L. (2008) *Could It Be Dementia?* Oxford: Monarch.

—— (2010) *Dementia: Frank and Linda's story.* Oxford: Monarch.

—— (2015) *Dementia: Pathways to Hope.* Oxford: Monarch.

—— (2010) *Worshipping with Dementia.* Oxford: Monarch.

Oxenham, J. (1852–1941) quotes can be found at: <http://izquotes.com/quote/348967>.

Procter, A. A. (1858) *Legends and Lyrics: A book of verse.* London: Bell & Daldy.

Stokes, Graham (2010) *And Still the Music Plays: Stories of people with dementia.* London: Hawker Publications.